YOU ARE

A SURVIVOR

In

CAROLYN McCLEAN

My grandmother talked to me a lot about what she called, life lessons. I made it my business to practice what she preached. She would say, "Lil girl in life you're gonna go through some stuff, always remember to stay in prayer because prayer changes things, Be good to yourself and others but, don't let nobody make an ass out of you and never take anyone or anything for granted because at a blink of an eye everything can change." On 3/26/2017, I Blinked.

LET ME EXPLAIN:
Saturday 3/25/2017: Woke up, got out of bed, brushed my teeth, had my daily talk with God, took a shower, made breakfast, spoke to friends and family, and went outside to run errands typical Saturday.

Sunday 3/26/2017: Woke up, got out of bed, brushed my teeth, had my daily talk with god, turned on some gospel music, made breakfast, cleaned my house, took a shower, went outside to do my taxes, watched tv, spoke to friends and family, Had A STROKE, A STROKE, I HAD A STROKE. Not my typical Sunday

Monday 3/27/2017: Woke up, and couldn't get out of the bed, I cried angrily, as I had my daily talk with God. I was full of uncontrollable emotions. I kept hearing my grandmother's words, " Don't take anyone or anything for granted." as I lay in a hospital bed reluctantly allowing a nurse to bathe me when it was all good just two days ago.

911: What's Your Emergency
ME: STROKE, STROKE, I'M HAVING A STROKE

CONVERSATION WITH SELF:
NO NO NO, I told myself this can't be happening screaming inside STOP! PLEASE STOP, PLEASE I pleaded with my brain but, it ignored my cry while trying to alter my speech and my movements it was separating from my body.
I kept screaming inside FIGHT BACK, IM SCARED PLEASE DON'T DO THIS TO ME, TO US. I was losing control and definitely having a stroke. At that moment my world changed.

What is my name:
The doctor asked me my name and I was not sure. God, please help me. I instantly began to cry. I hesitantly guessed, "Carolyn" looking over at my daughter for reassurance speaking with my eyes "Am I right, Please say I'm right"

Testimony:
Today when I tell people that I had a stroke, they look at me with disbelief. Most would say, " You don't look like you had a stroke."
I simply smile and say, "Yes I did, actually I had two along with a small bleed in my brain caused by the medication given to me to stop the stroke from causing more damage. I know that part sounds ironic and you may not understand but, to be able to articulate the words " I Am A Stroke Survivor" is a blessing to me because I know the outcome could have been different. Maybe I would not have survived to tell this story or perhaps I would be sitting before you not being able to walk or speak at all." There are pieces of me that I don't think I'll get back. I function a little differently, my thought pattern is a little different but, without hesitation or reassurance I know my name is CAROLYN JOYCE MCCLEAN
I am A Stroke Survivor.

As my grandmother always said, there is no medicine like gods medicine, and prayer changes things. I am ever so grateful to my family and friends for all the love and prayers that continuously shower over me. THANK YOU to my daughters Tiffany and Tiggy. It was you two that called grandma Primes for that extra special prayer as I lay in that hospital bed almost facing death. I know without a shadow of a doubt that her prayer to God saved my life that night and made it possible to tell my story today.

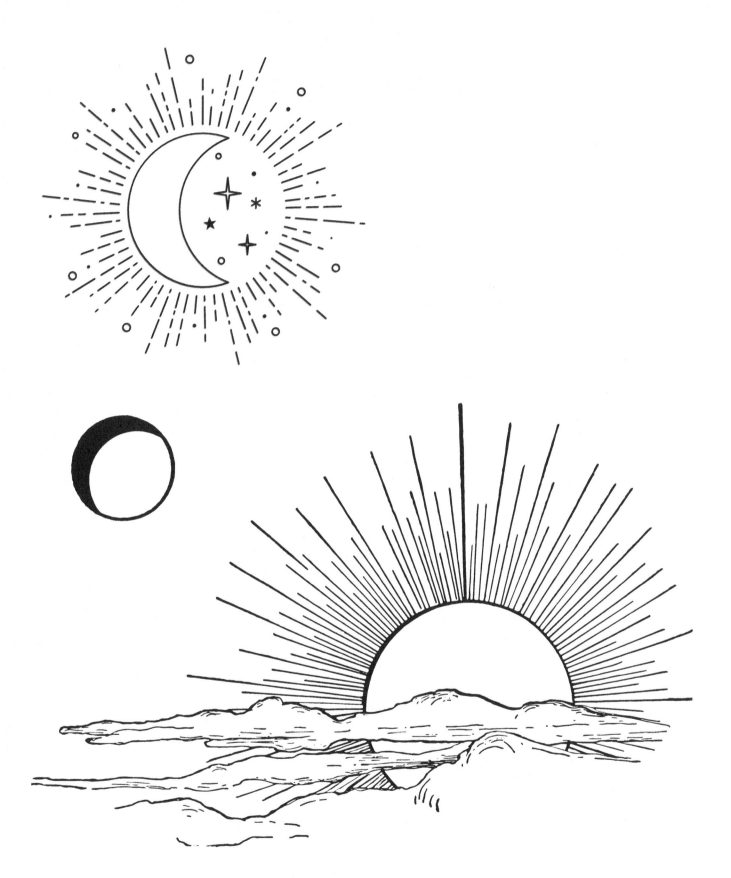

Fruit That Starts With B

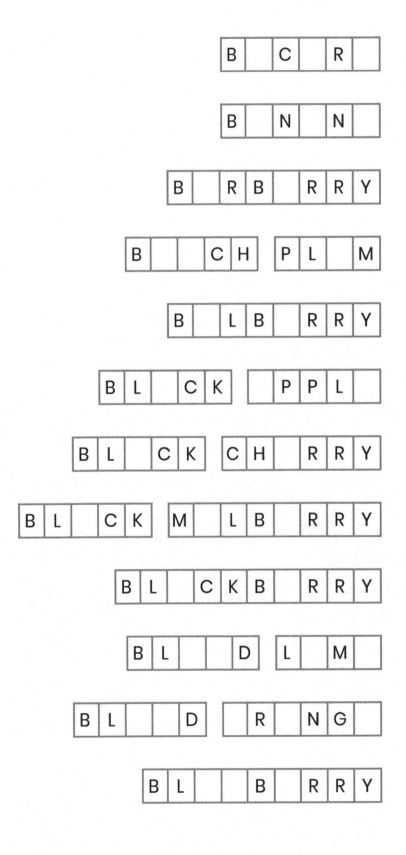

Fruit That Starts With B - Solution

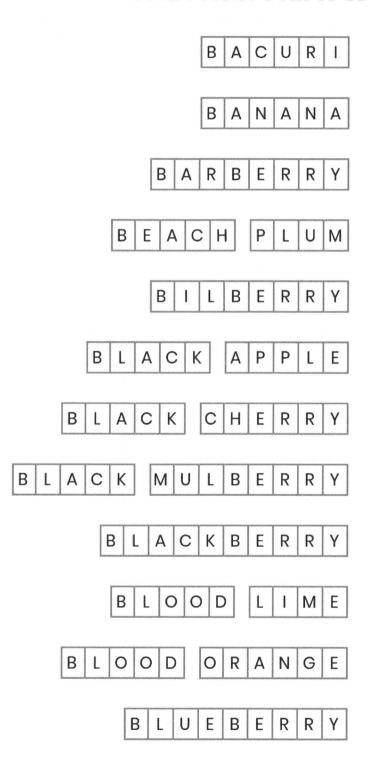

B A C U R I

B A N A N A

B A R B E R R Y

B E A C H   P L U M

B I L B E R R Y

B L A C K   A P P L E

B L A C K   C H E R R Y

B L A C K   M U L B E R R Y

B L A C K B E R R Y

B L O O D   L I M E

B L O O D   O R A N G E

B L U E B E R R Y

Fruit That Start With P

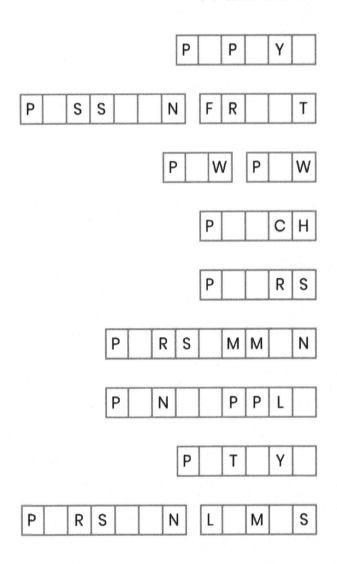

Fruit That Start With P – Solution

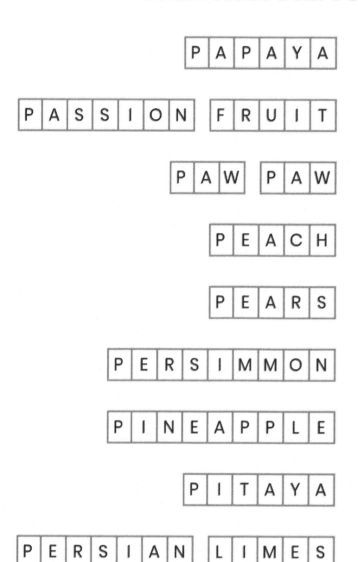

PAPAYA

PASSION FRUIT

PAW PAW

PEACH

PEARS

PERSIMMON

PINEAPPLE

PITAYA

PERSIAN LIMES

Fruit That Start With O

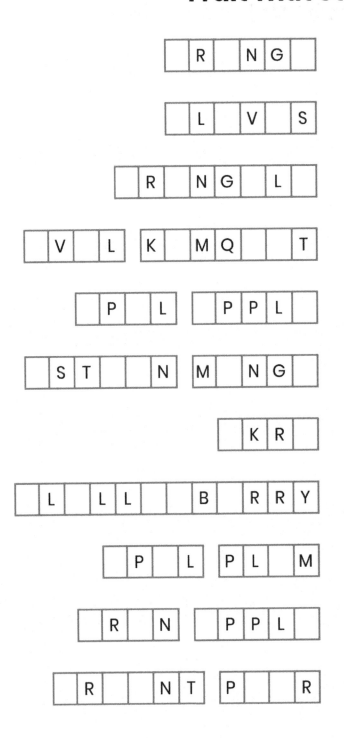

```
_ R _ N G _

_ L _ V _ S

_ R _ N G _ L _

_ V _ L _ K _ M Q _ _ T

_ P _ L   _ P P L _

_ S T _ _ N   M _ N G _

_ K R _

_ L _ L L _ _ B _ R R Y

_ P _ L   P _ L M

_ R _ N   P P L _

_ R _ N T P _ _ R
```

Fruit That Start With O - Solution

ORANGE

OLIVES

ORANGELO

OVAL KUMQUAT

OPAL APPLE

OSTEEN MANGO

OKRA

OLALLIEBERRY

OPAL PLUM

ORIN APPLE

OREINT PEAR

Don't Touch Without Asking Me First

ARC ☐☐☐

DKI ☐☐☐

TPE ☐☐☐

YMEON ☐☐☐☐☐

ETEF ☐☐☐☐

AIRH ☐☐☐☐

TPEMRTRUAEE SNIETTG ☐☐☐☐☐☐☐☐☐☐ ☐☐☐☐☐☐☐

PRMEFUE ☐☐☐☐☐☐☐

CTRALYSS ☐☐☐☐☐☐☐☐☐

YM YDBO ☐☐ ☐☐☐☐

RIAOTEGRERFR ☐☐☐☐☐☐☐☐☐☐☐☐☐

INEW ☐☐☐☐

CEEARL ☐☐☐☐☐☐

Don't Touch Without Asking Me First - Solution

ARC | C A R

DKI | K I D

TPE | P E T

YMEON | M O N E Y

ETEF | F E E T

AIRH | H A I R

TPEMRTRUAEE SNIETTG | T E M P E R A T U R E S E T T I N G

PRMEFUE | P E R F U M E

CTRALYSS | C R Y S T A L S

YM YDBO | M Y B O D Y

RIAOTEGRERFR | R E F R I G E R A T O R

INEW | W I N E

CEEARL | C E R E A L

Things That Smell Over Time

UMERNRADS [ ][ ][ ][ ][ ][ ][ ][ ][ ]

BTREAH [ ][ ][ ][ ][ ][ ]

IFRTU [ ][ ][ ][ ][ ]

ATEM [ ][ ][ ][ ]

TBUT [ ][ ][ ][ ]

EETF [ ][ ][ ][ ]

ARHI [ ][ ][ ][ ]

LMKI [ ][ ][ ][ ]

GDO [ ][ ][ ]

AUDTTITE [ ][ ][ ][ ][ ][ ][ ][ ]

Things That Smell Over Time - Solution

UMERNRADS | U N D E R A R M S

BTREAH | B R E A T H

IFRTU | F R U I T

ATEM | M E A T

TBUT | B U T T

EETF | F E E T

ARHI | H A I R

LMKI | M I L K

GDO | D O G

AUDTTITE | A T T I T U D E

Things You Like

WSLO SMJA ☐☐☐☐ ☐☐☐☐

XSE ☐☐

LONEA MEIT ☐☐☐☐☐ ☐☐☐☐

DCINANG ☐☐☐☐☐☐

FLGO ☐☐☐

INOBG ☐☐☐☐

SEIPNLEG ☐☐☐☐☐☐☐

GAOY ☐☐☐

BSBTAAKLEL ☐☐☐☐☐☐☐☐☐☐

TNINANG ☐☐☐☐☐☐

ETNAIG ☐☐☐☐☐

LFOG ☐☐☐

Things You Like - Solution

WSLO SMJA S L O W   J A M S

XSE S E X

LONEA MEIT A L O N E   T I M E

DCINANG D A N C I N G

FLGO G O L F

INOBG B I N G O

SEIPNLEG S L E E P I N G

GAOY Y O G A

BSBTAAKLEL B A S K E T B A L L

TNINANG T A N N I N G

ETNAIG E A T I N G

LFOG G O L F

Things You May Dislike

PCHA IPSL □□□□ □□□□

OUDL THOUM □□□□ □□□□□

SPKIINPG HET NLEI □□□□□□□□ □□□□ □□□□□

ASG PCREIS □□□ □□□□□□

ETH DCOL □□□ □□□□

GBEIN NA UTDAL □□□□□ □□ □□□□□

DEISHS NI INKS □□□□□□ □□ □□□□

OURY SDKI □□□□ □□□□

USBG □□□□

DIERVRS □□□□□□□

Things You May Dislike - Solution

PCHA IPSL — C H A P   L I P S

OUDL THOUM — L O U D   M O U T H

SPKIINPG HET NLEI — S K I P P I N G   T H E   L I N E

ASG PCREIS — G A S   P R I C E S

ETH DCOL — T H E   C O L D

GBEIN NA UTDAL — B E I N G   A N   A D U L T

DEISHS NI INKS — D I S H E S   I N   S I N K

OURY SDKI — Y O U R   K I D S

USBG — B U G S

DIERVRS — D R I V E R S

US Department Stores

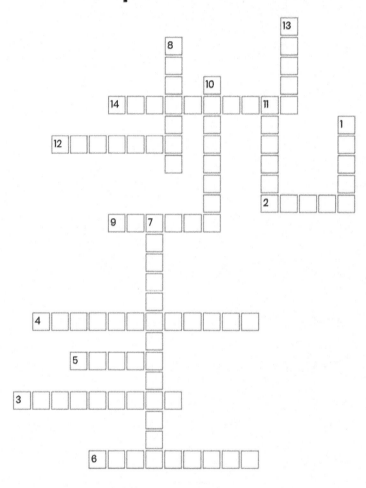

<table>
<tr><td>

Across

[2]

[3]

[4]

[5]

[6]

[9]

[12]

[14]

</td><td>

Down

[1]

[7]

[8]

[10]

[11]

[13]

</td></tr>
</table>

US Department Stores - Solution

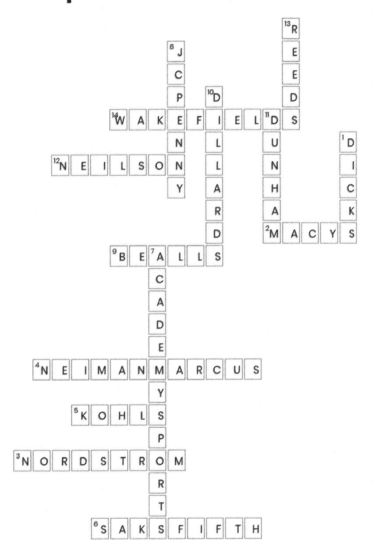

Summer Time

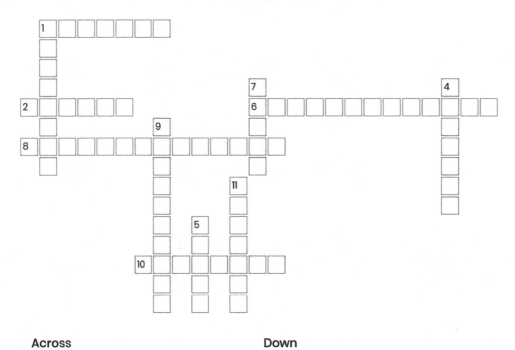

Across
[1]
[2]
[6]
[8]
[10]

Down
[1]
[4]
[5]
[7]
[9]
[11]

Summer Time - Solution

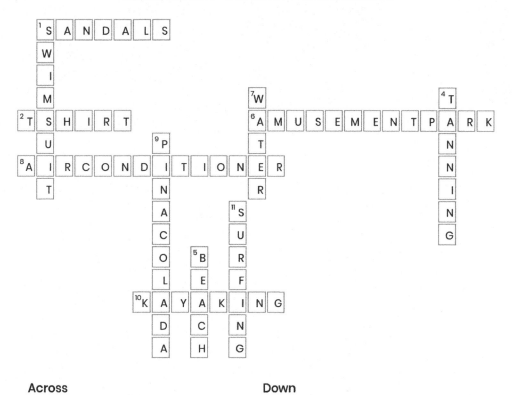

Across
[1]
[2]
[6]
[8]
[10]

Down
[1]
[4]
[5]
[7]
[9]
[11]

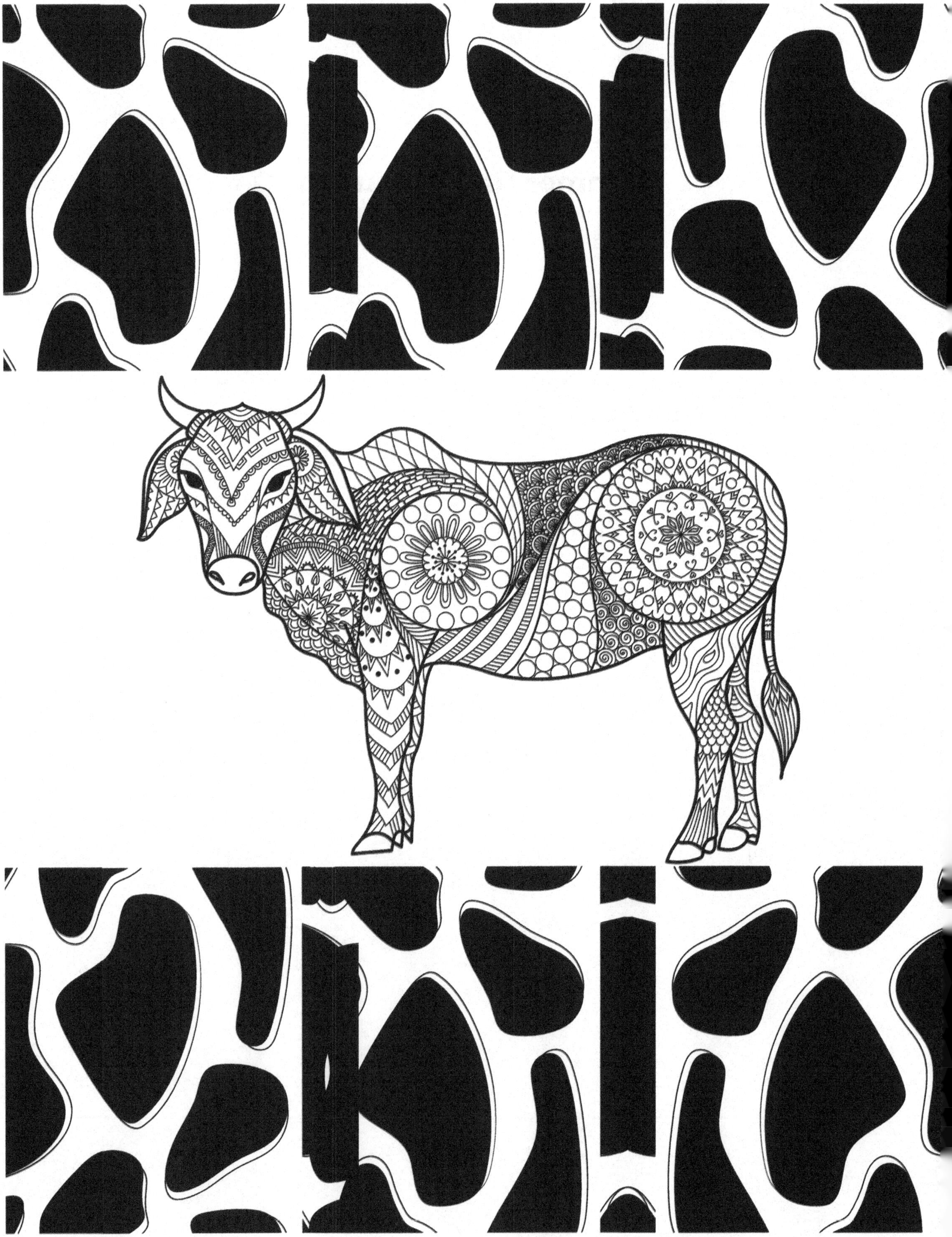

Top Beaches

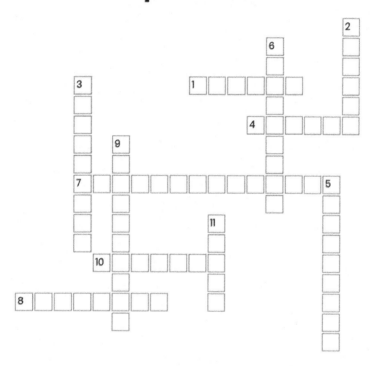

Across
[1]

[4]

[7]

[8]

[10]

Down
[2]

[3]

[5]

[6]

[9]

[11]

Top Beaches - Solution

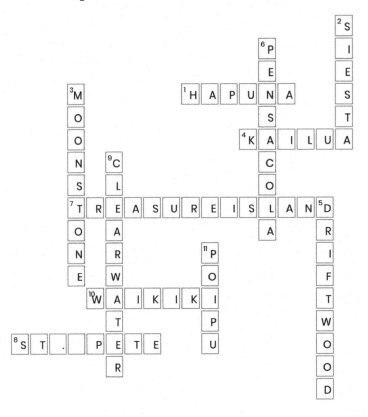

Across

[1]

[4]

[7]

[8]

[10]

Down

[2]

[3]

[5]

[6]

[9]

[11]

Snacks

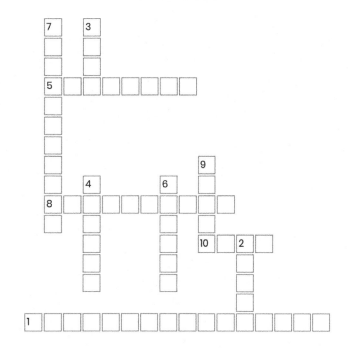

Across
[1]

[5]

[8]

[10]

Down
[2]

[3]

[4]

[6]

[7]

[9]

Snacks - Solution

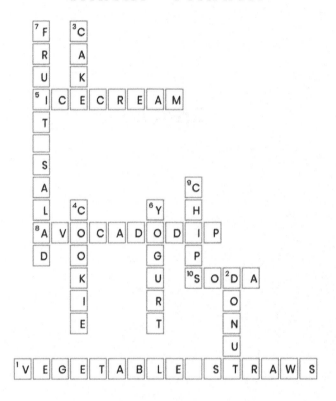

Across

[1]

[5]

[8]

[10]

Down

[2]

[3]

[4]

[6]

[7]

[9]

Foreign Cars

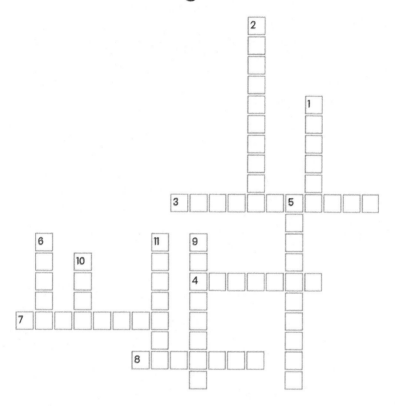

Across
[3]
[4]
[7]
[8]

Down
[1]
[2]
[5]
[6]
[9]
[10]
[11]

Foreign Cars - Solution

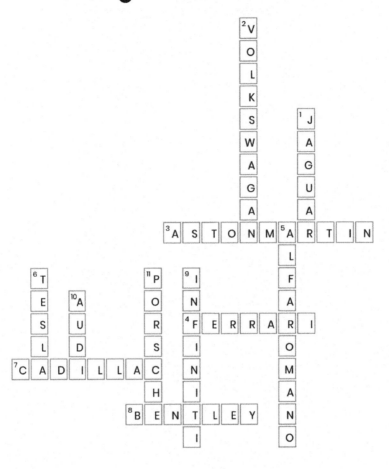

Across

[3]

[4]

[7]

[8]

Down

[1]

[2]

[5]

[6]

[9]

[10]

[11]

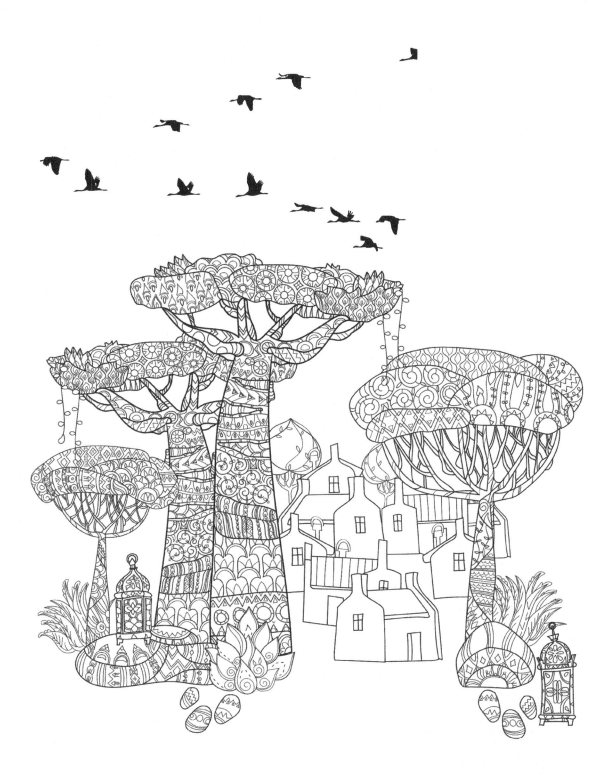

MAZE TIME

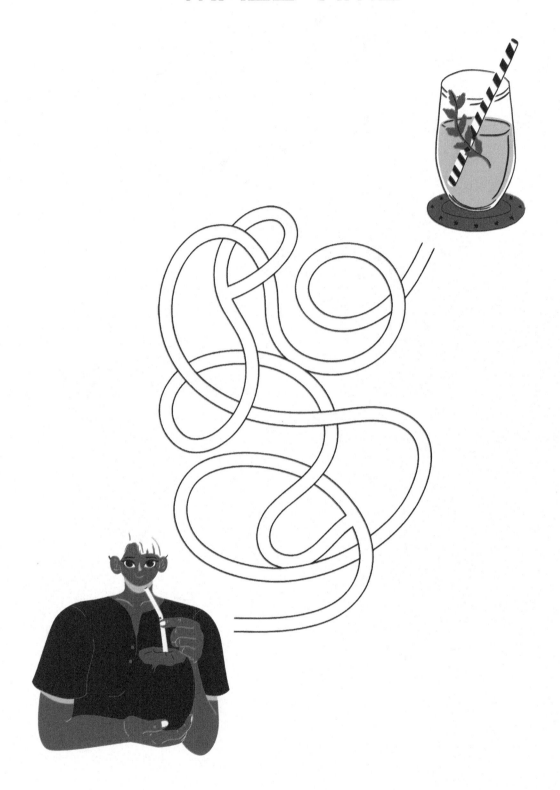

MAZE TIME

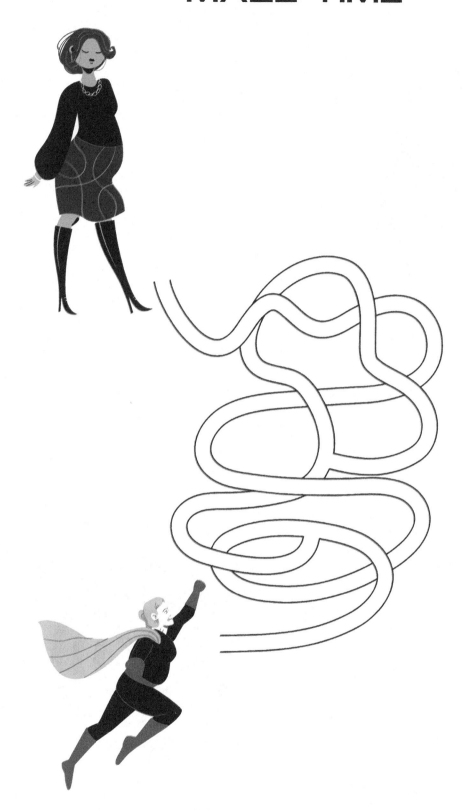

MAZE TIME

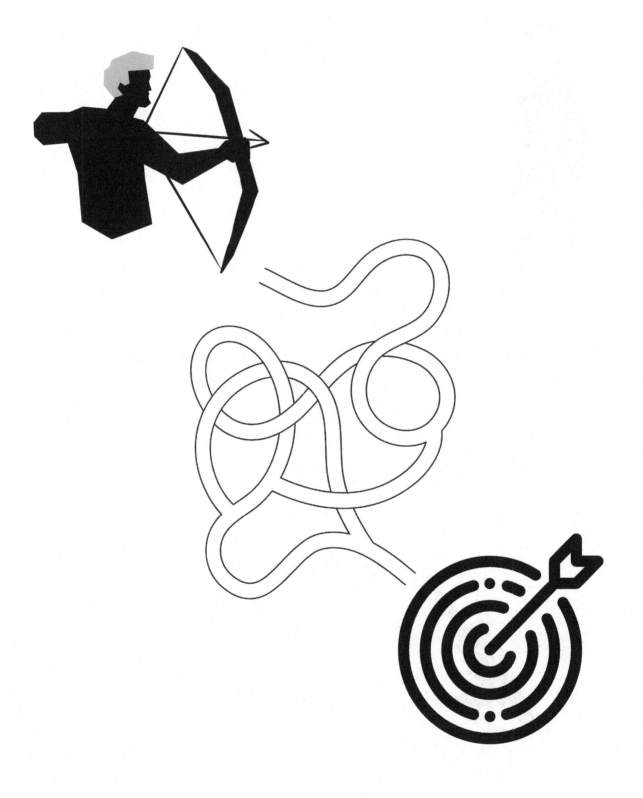

MAZE TIME

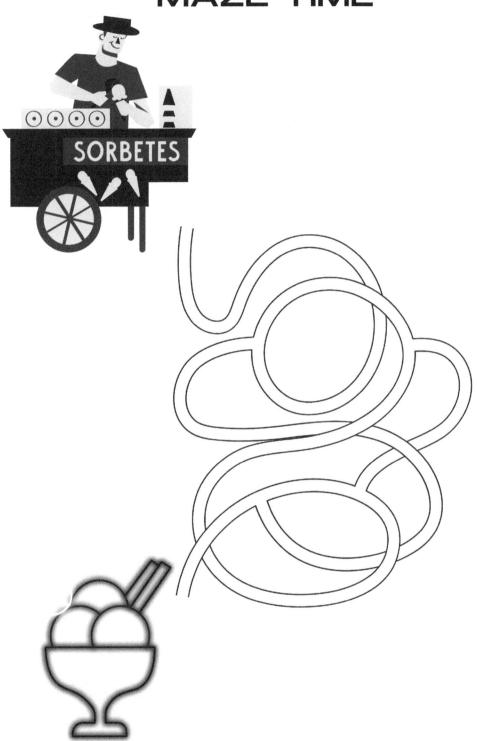

MAZE TIME

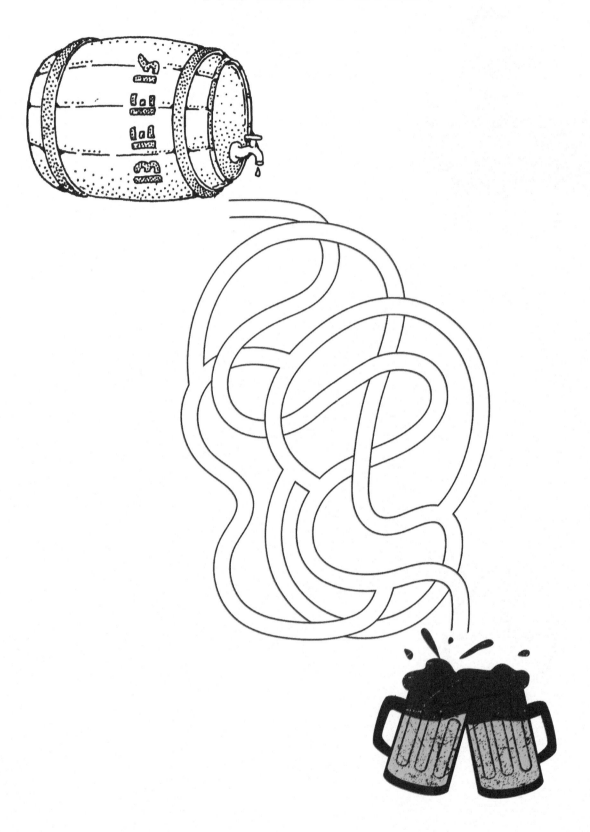

MAZE TIME

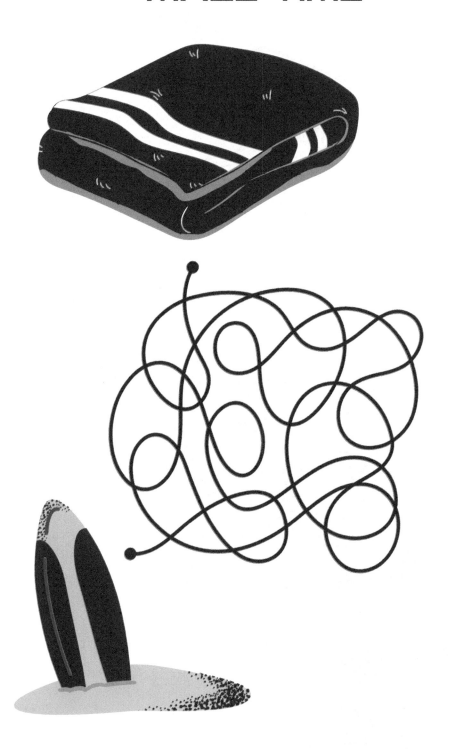

MAZE TIME

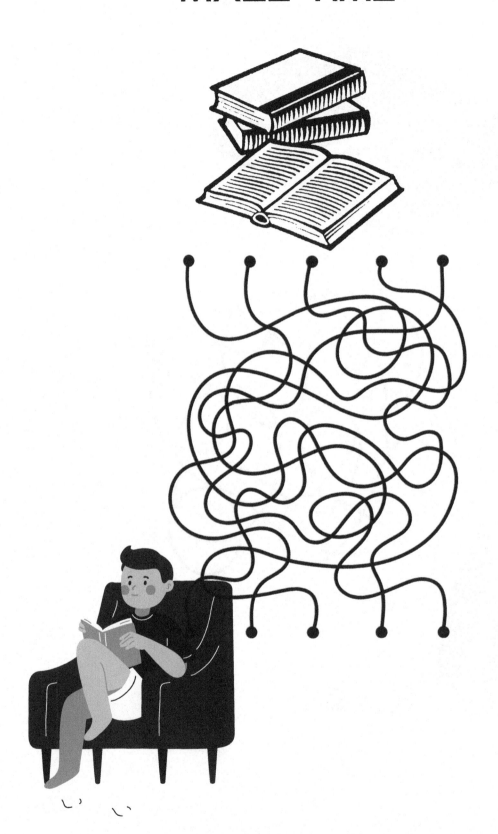

MAZE TIME

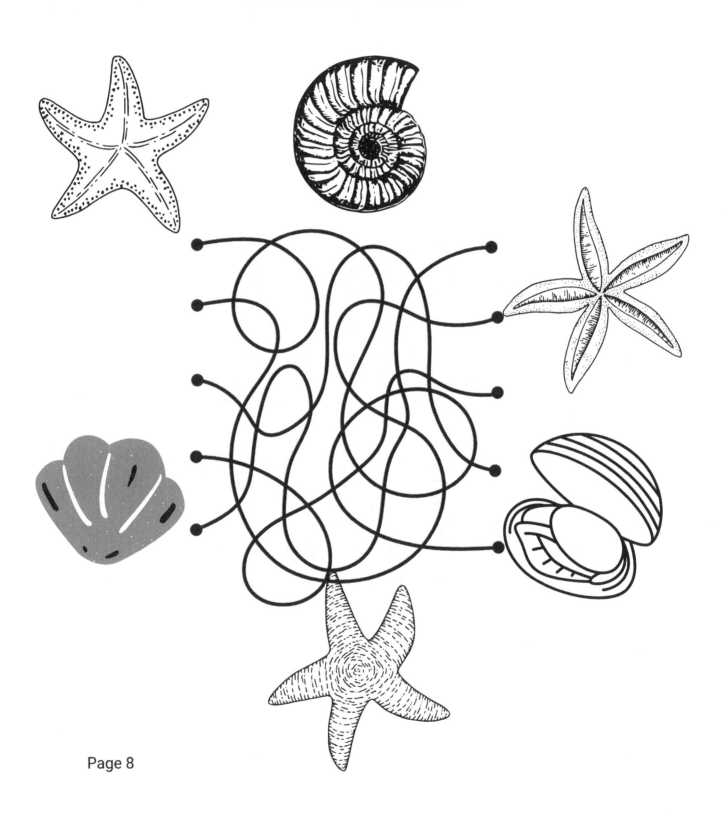

MAZE TIME

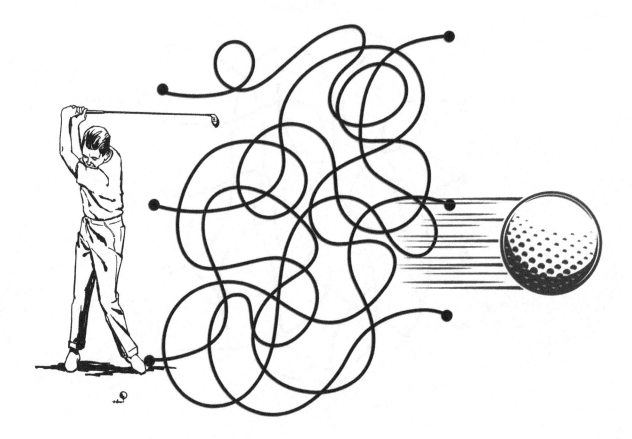

MAZE TIME

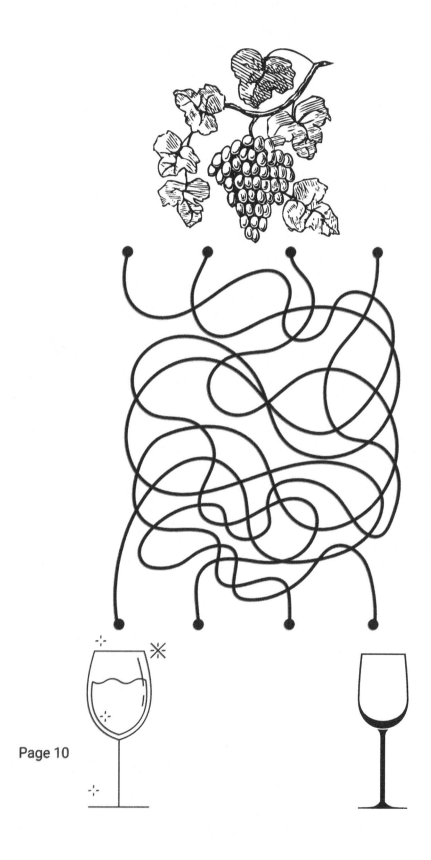

MAZE TIME

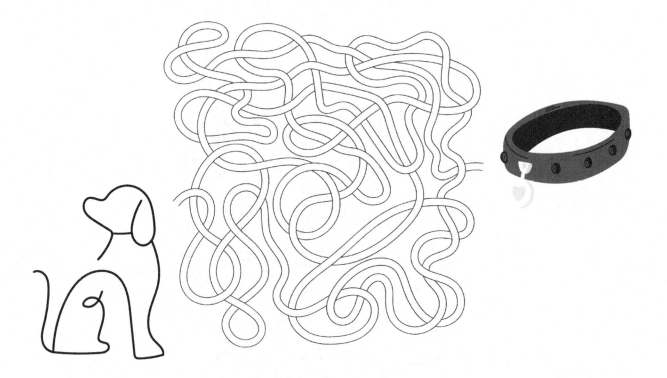

MAZE TIME

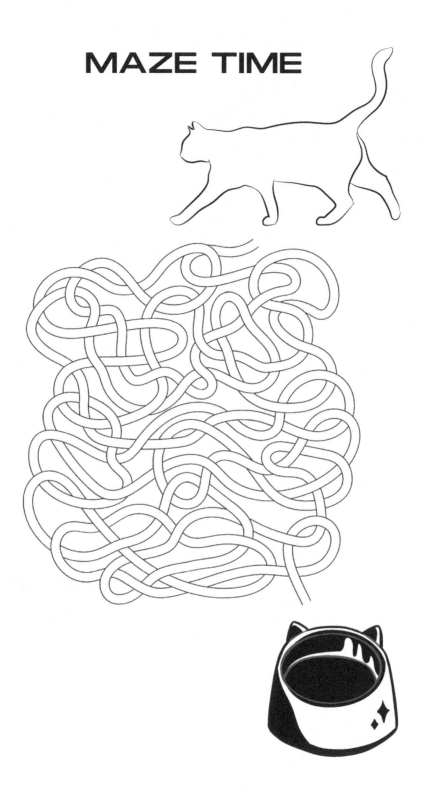

MAZE TIME

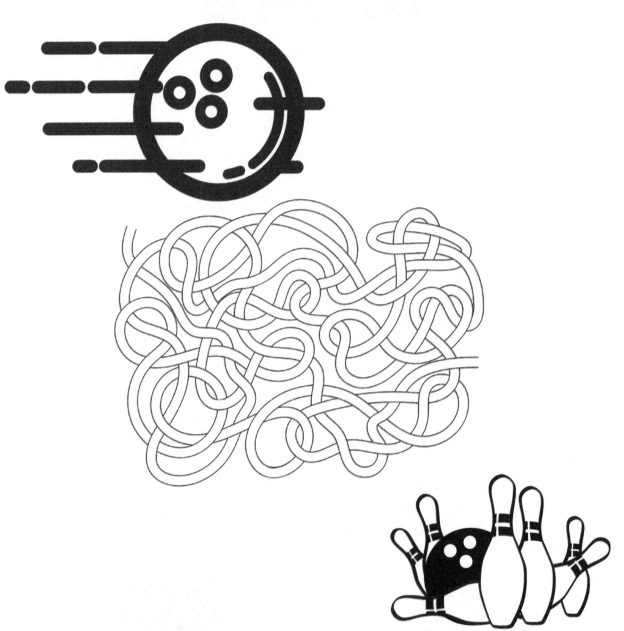

MAZE TIME

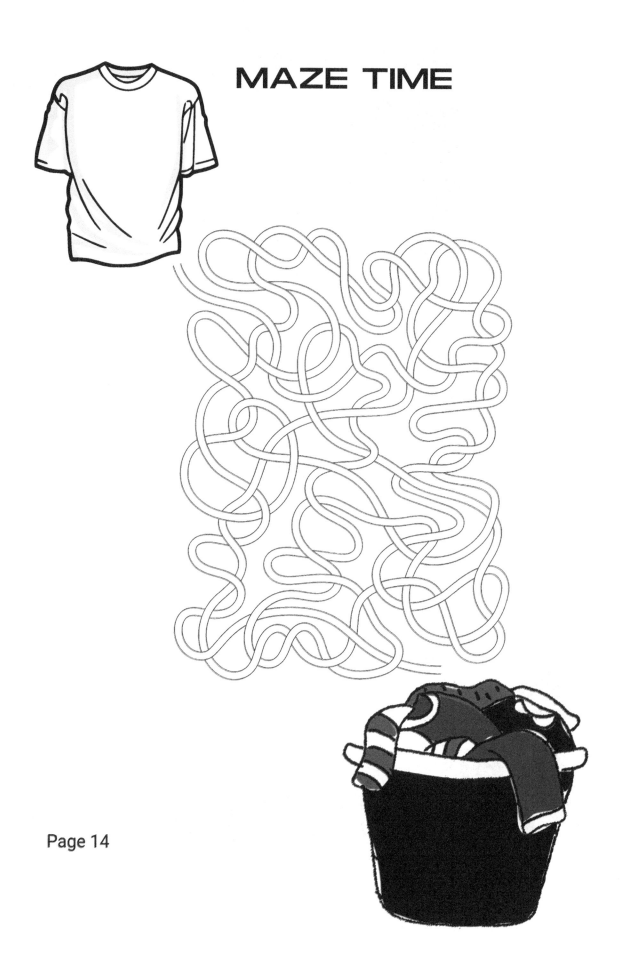

MAZE TIME

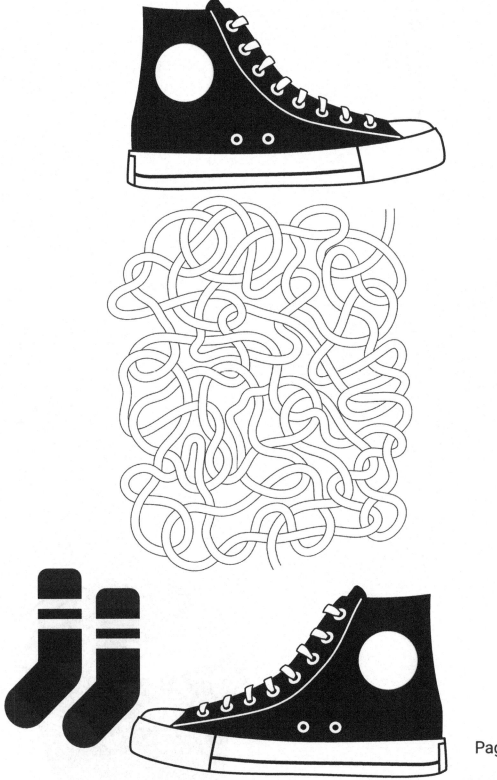

MAZE TIME

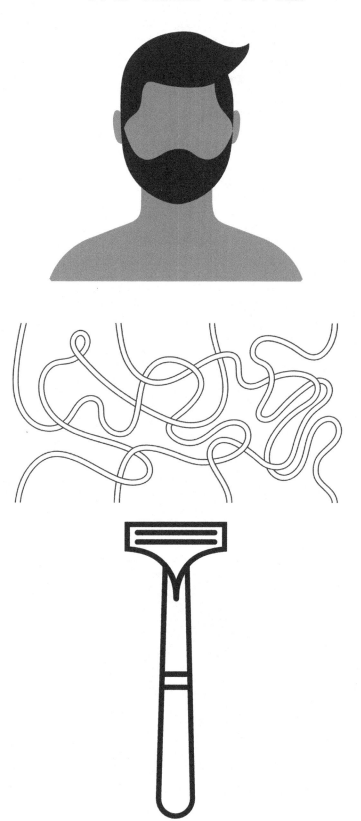

MAZE TIME

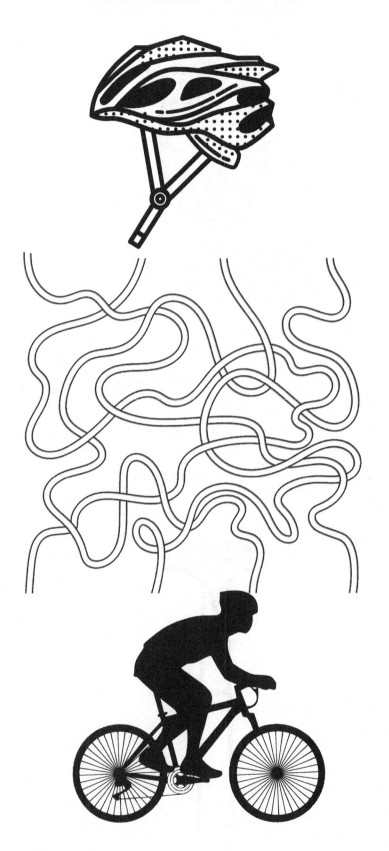

MAZE TIME

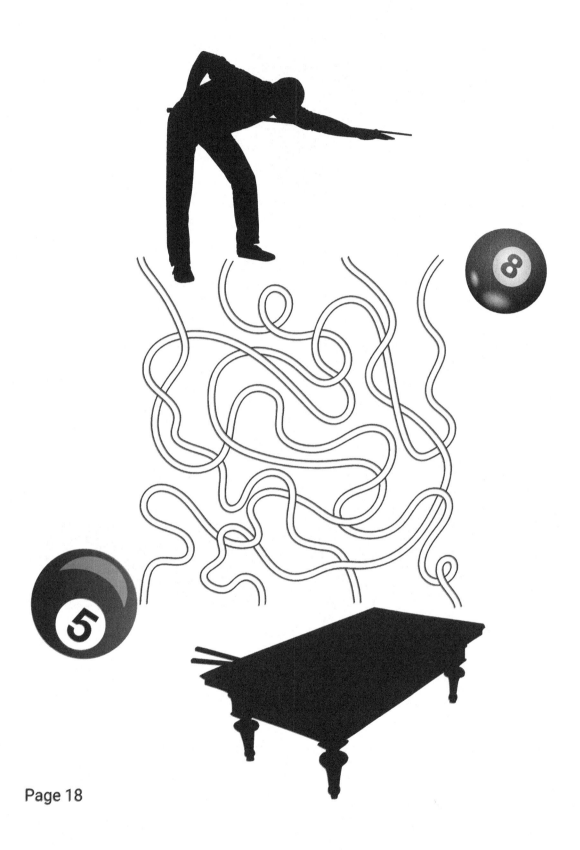

MAZE TIME

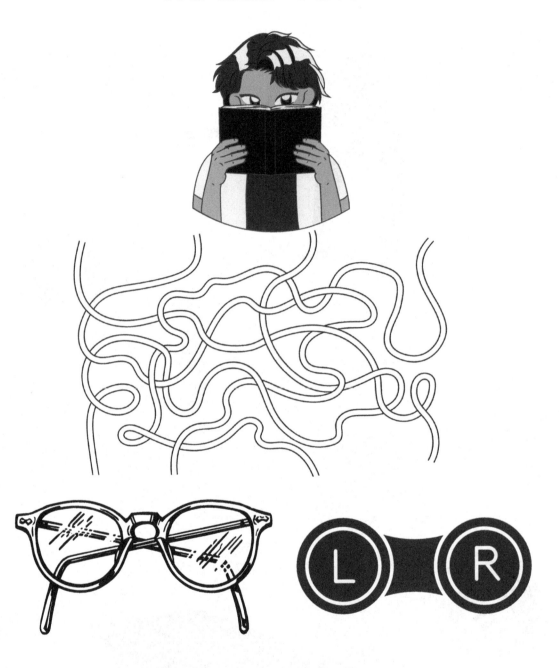

MAZE TIME

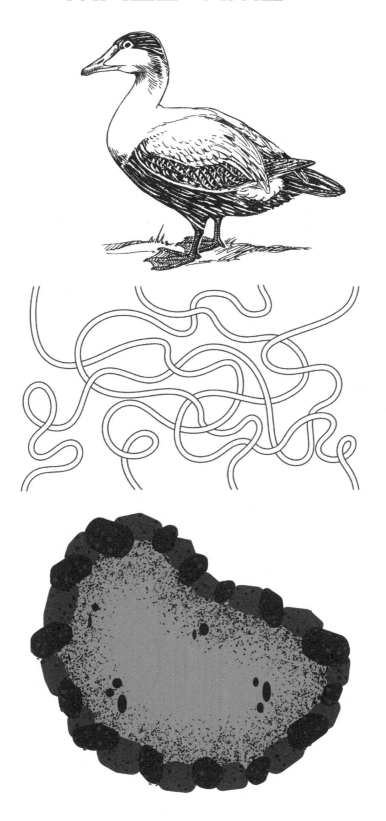

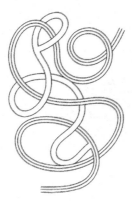

Page 1-1

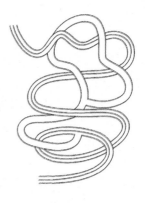

Page 2-1

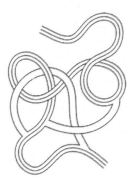

Page 3-1

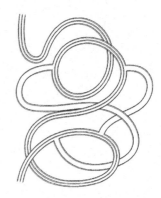

Page 4-1

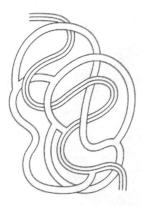

Page 5-1

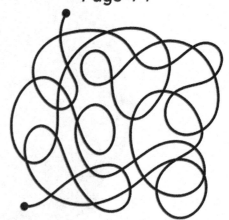

Page 6-1

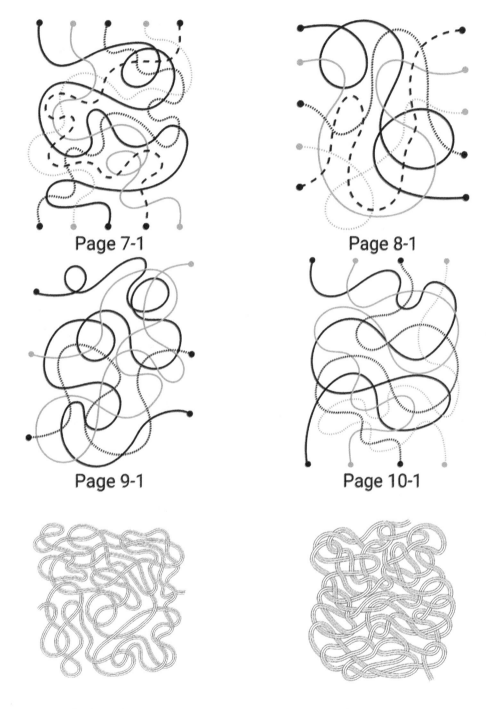

Page 7-1

Page 8-1

Page 9-1

Page 10-1

Page 11-1

Page 12-1

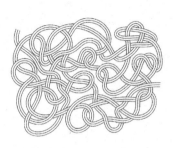

Page 13-1

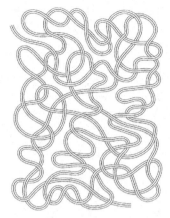

Page 14-1

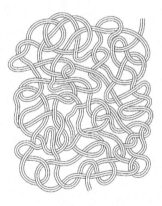

Page 15-1

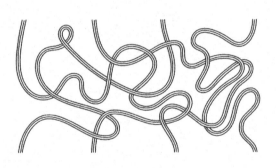

Page 16-1

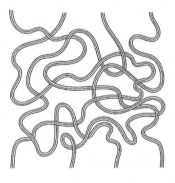

Page 17-1

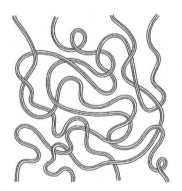

Page 18-1

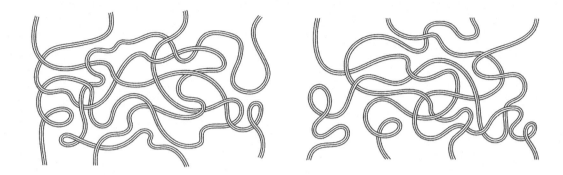

Page 19-1   Page 20-1

Trace

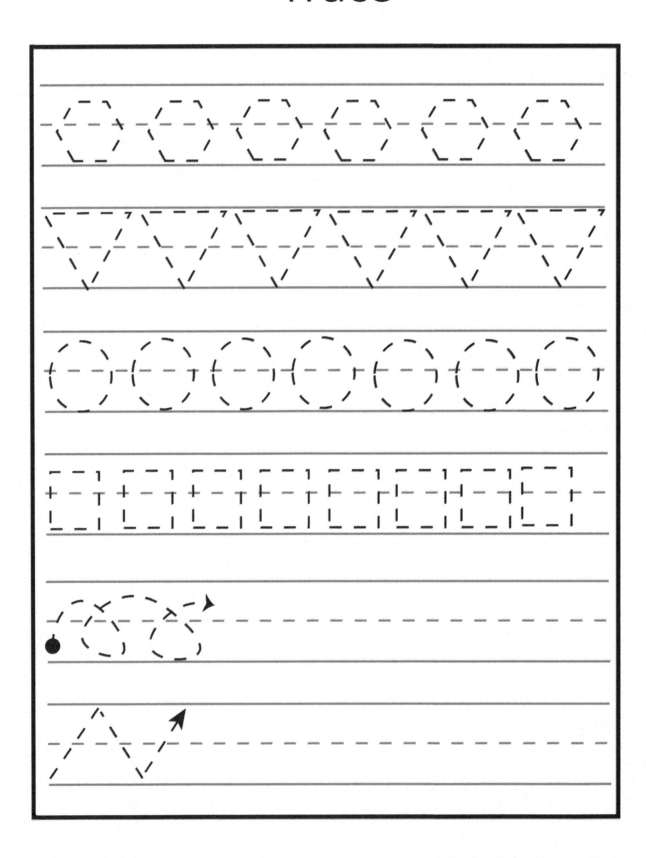

Trace The dotted Lines

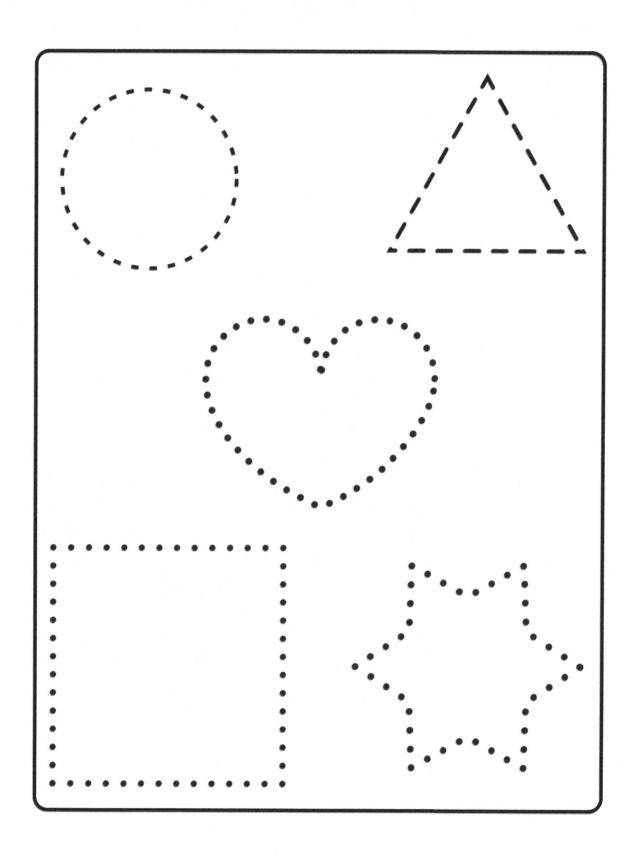

Color Me

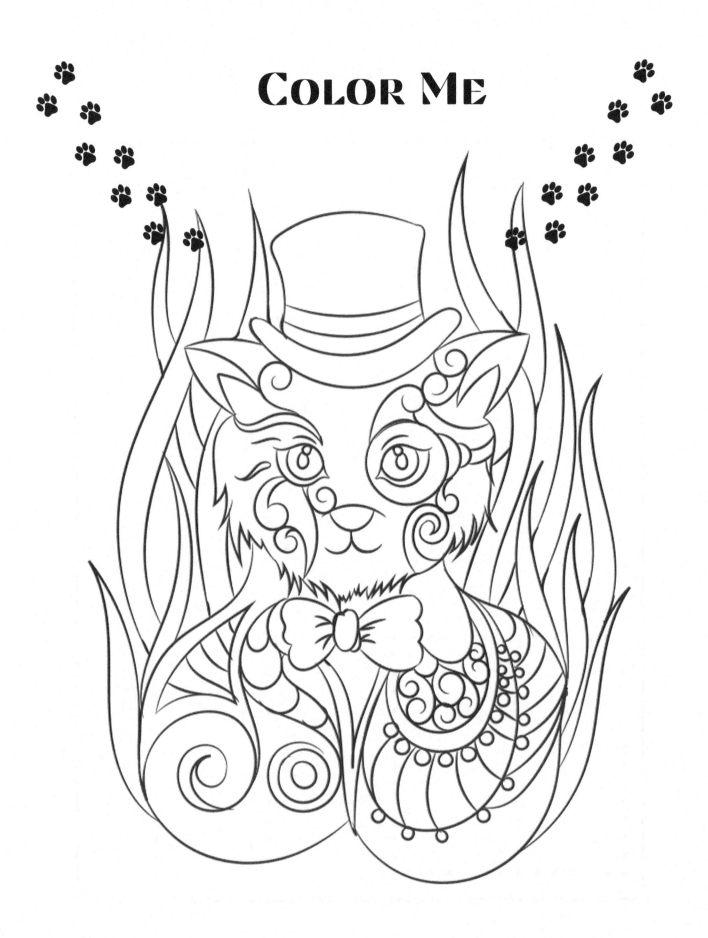

Color Me

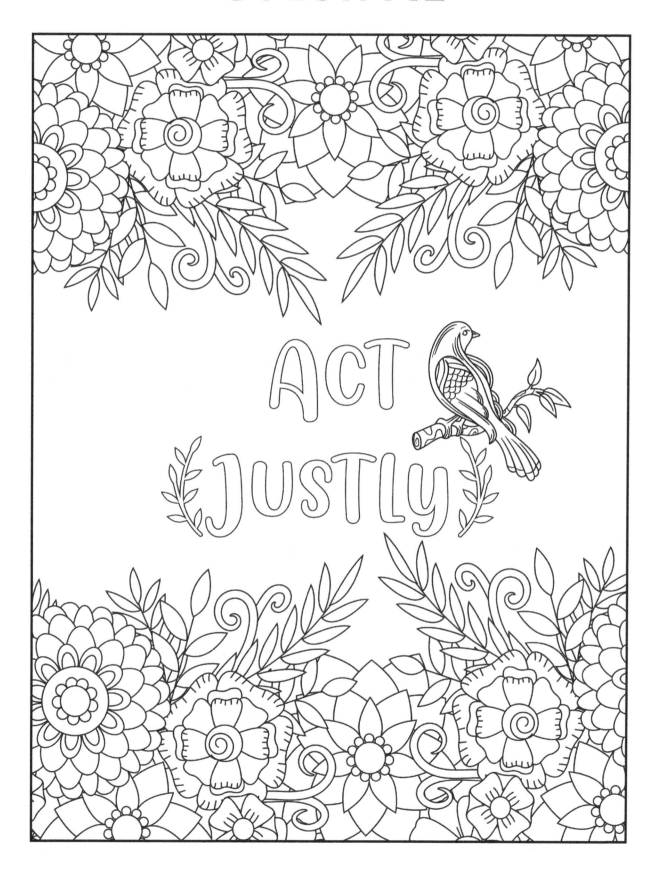

COLOR ME

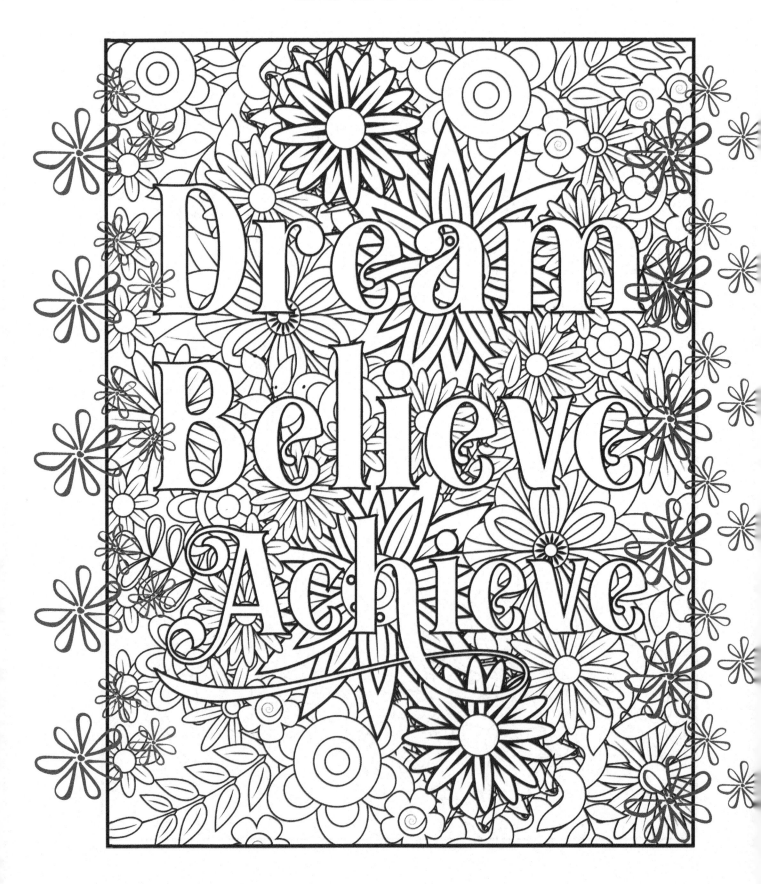

COLOR ME

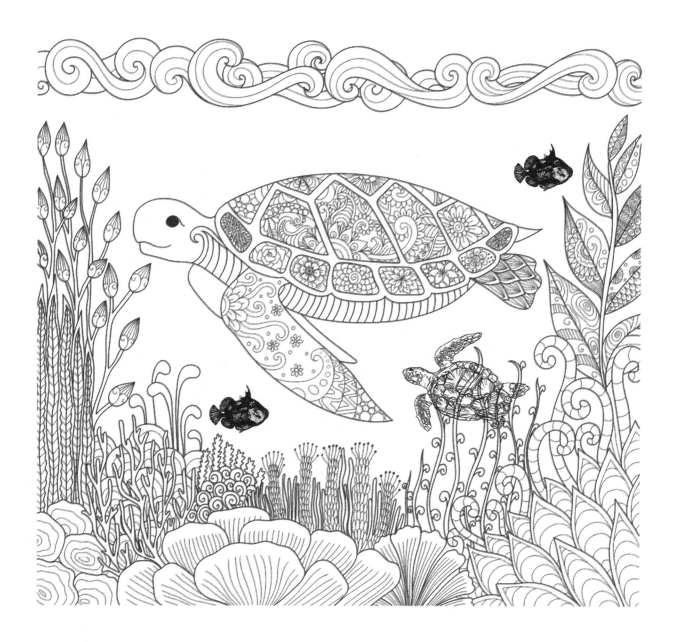

COLOR ME

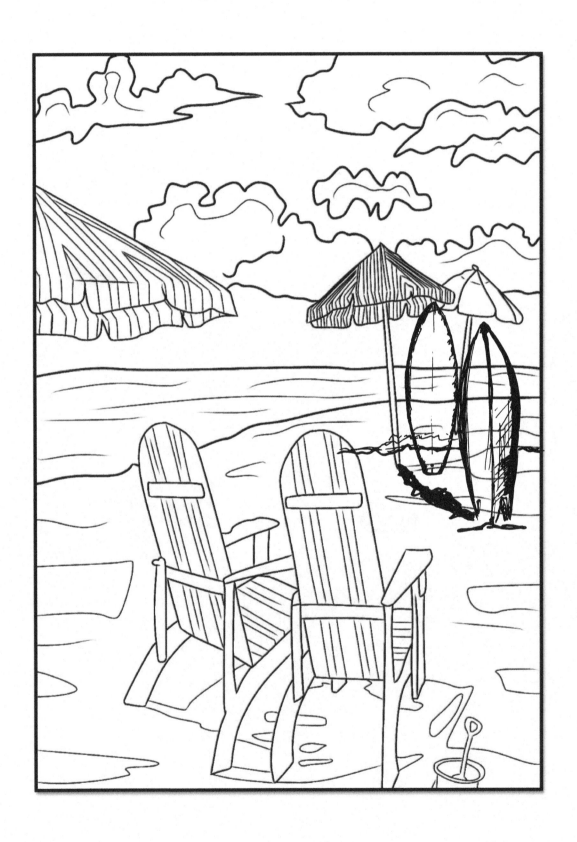

COLOR ME

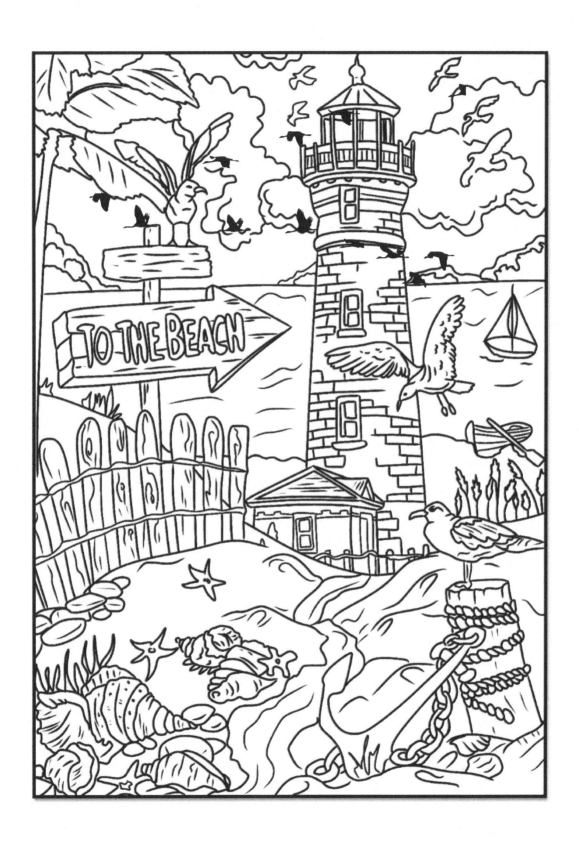

TRACE AND COLOR

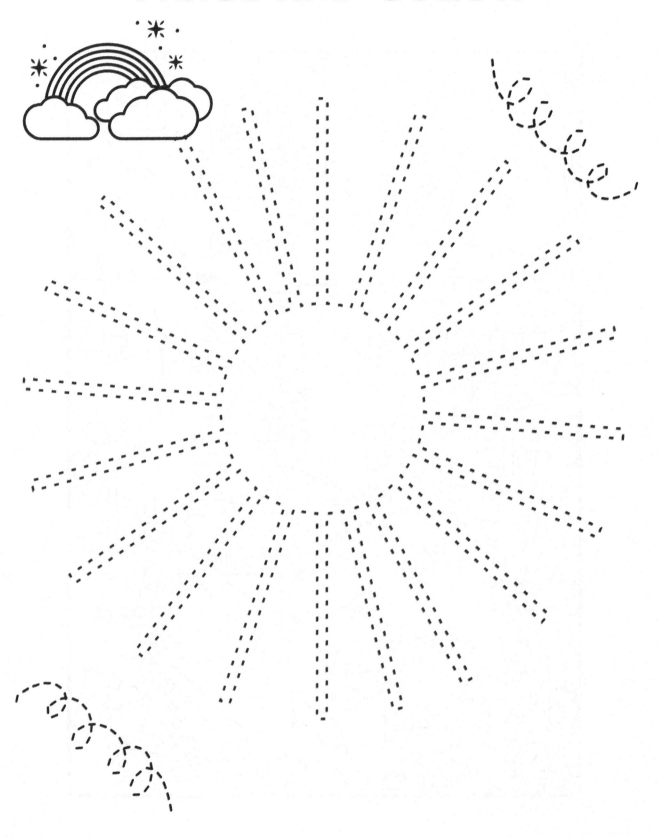

TRACE AND COLOR

SOCCER BALL

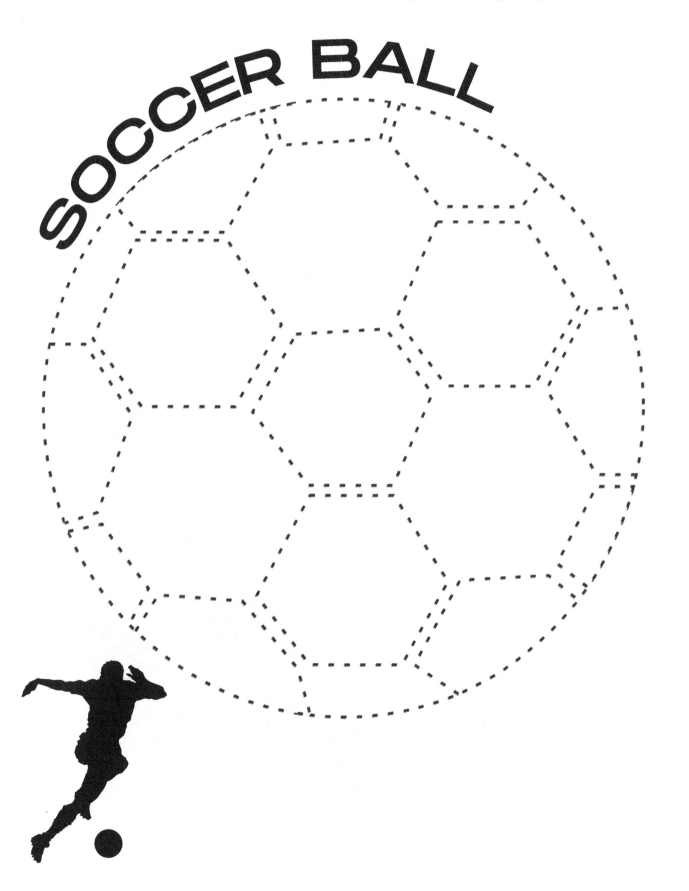

TRACE AND COLOR

LEAF

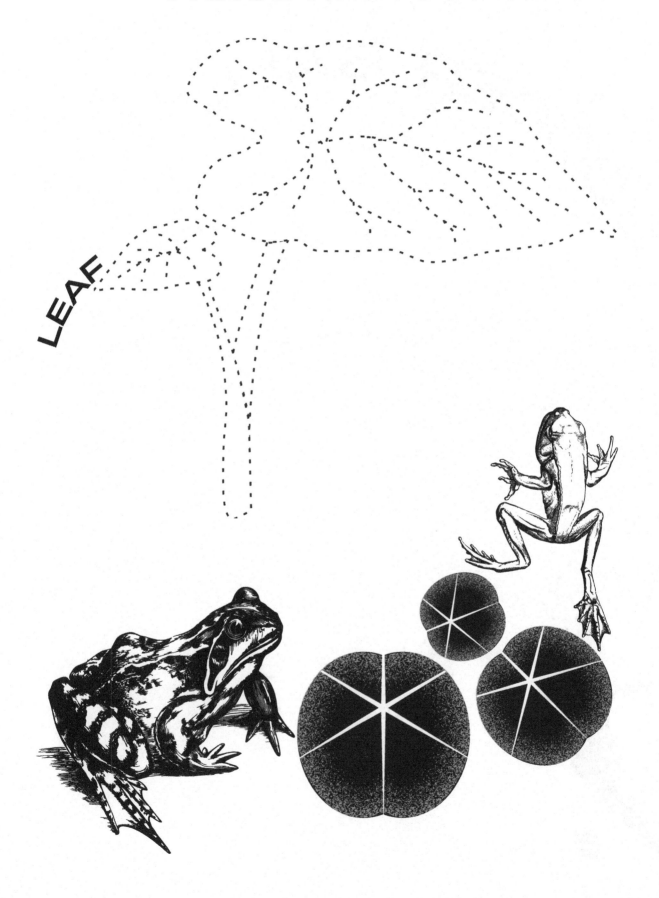

TRACE AND COLOR

BIRD

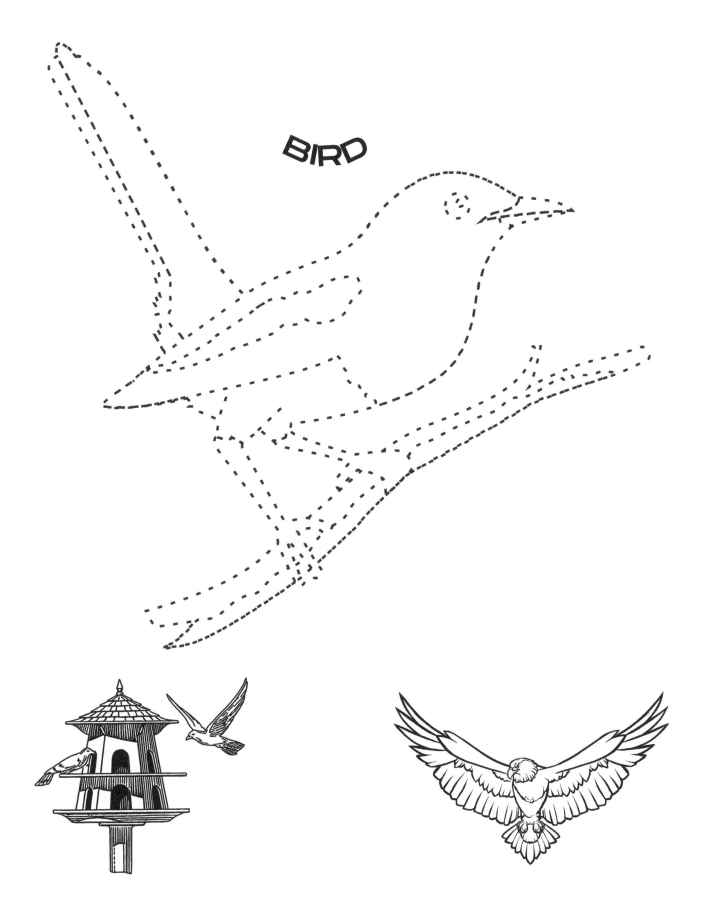

TRACE AND COLOR

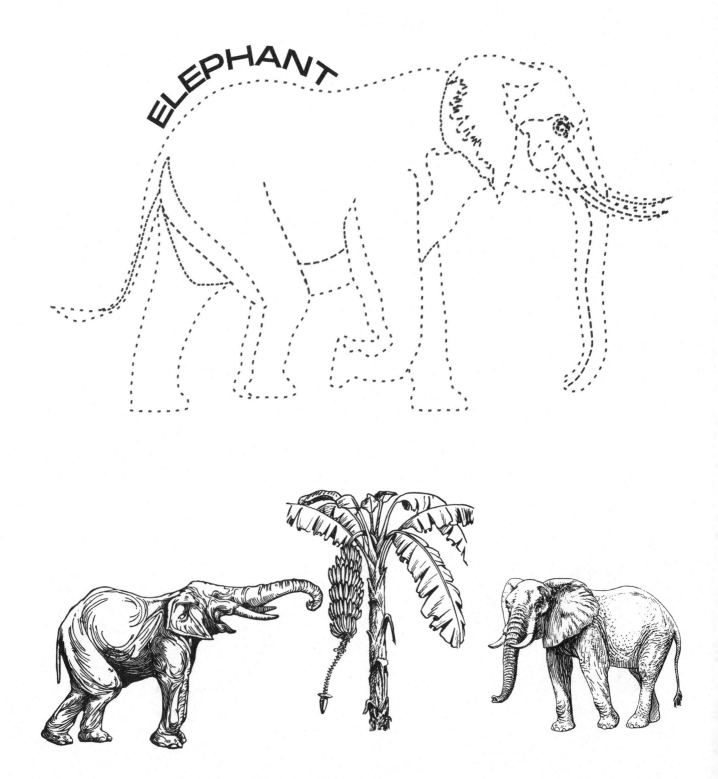

ELEPHANT

TRACE AND COLOR

TOMATO

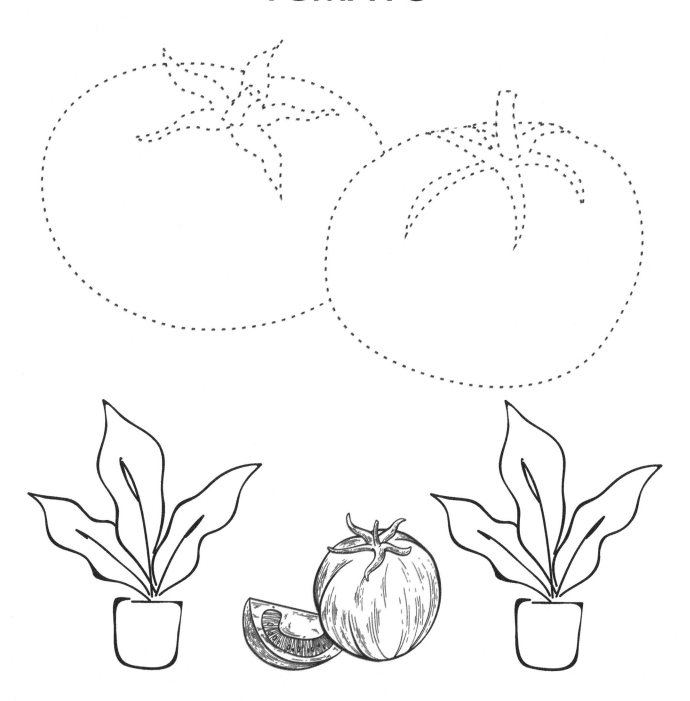

TRACE AND COLOR

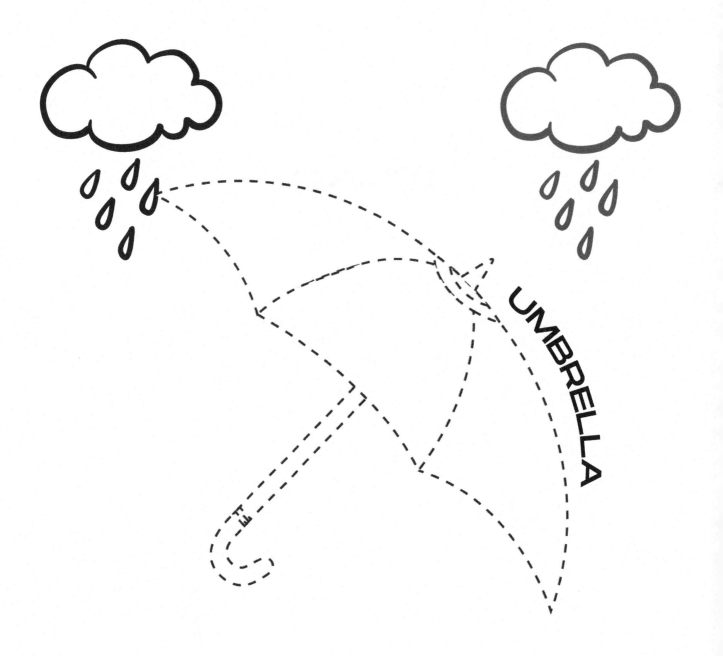

DRAW LINE AND MATCH COLORS

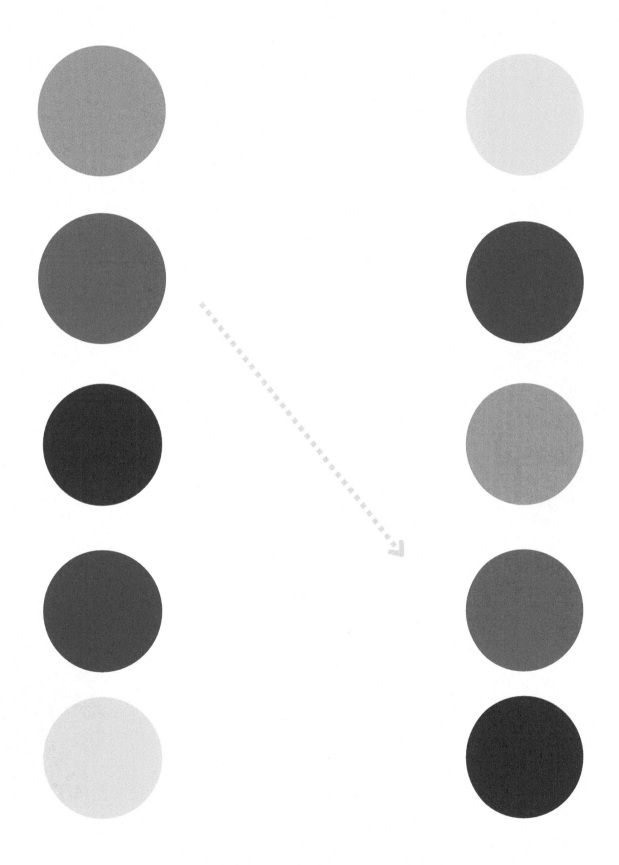

DRAW LINE AND MATCH COLOR

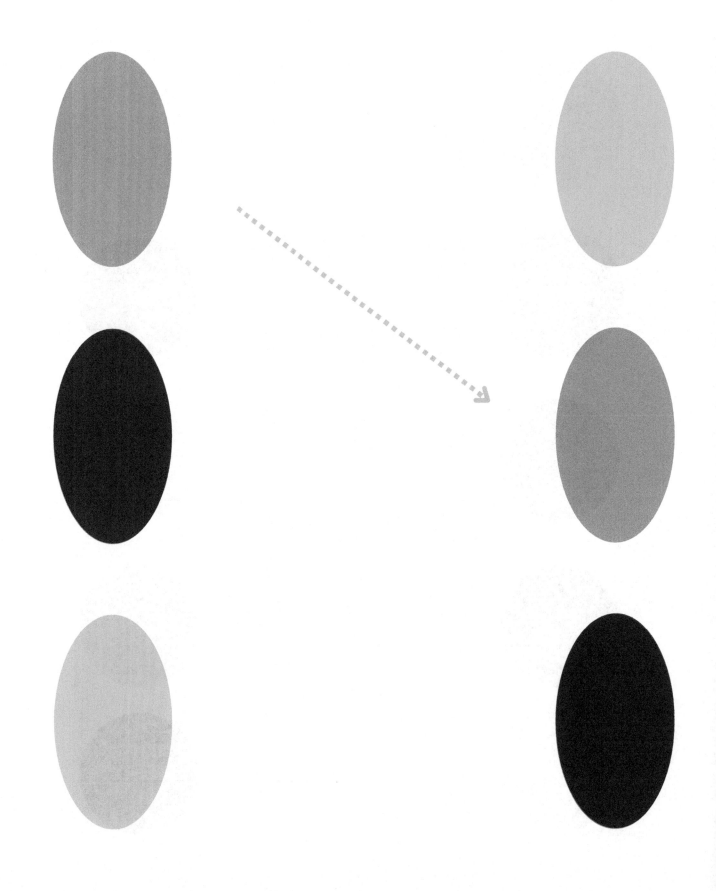

DRAW LINE AND MATCH COLOR

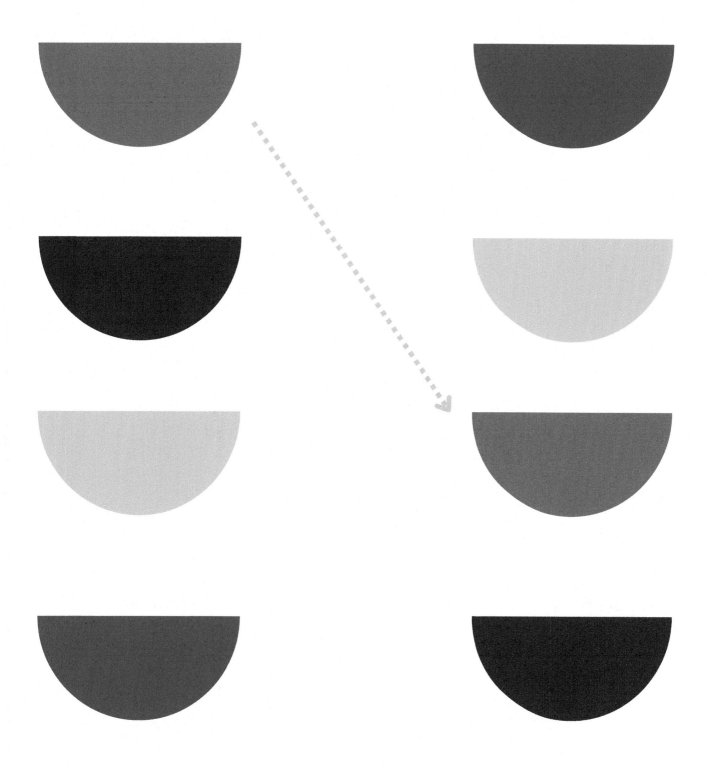

TRACE CIRCLES

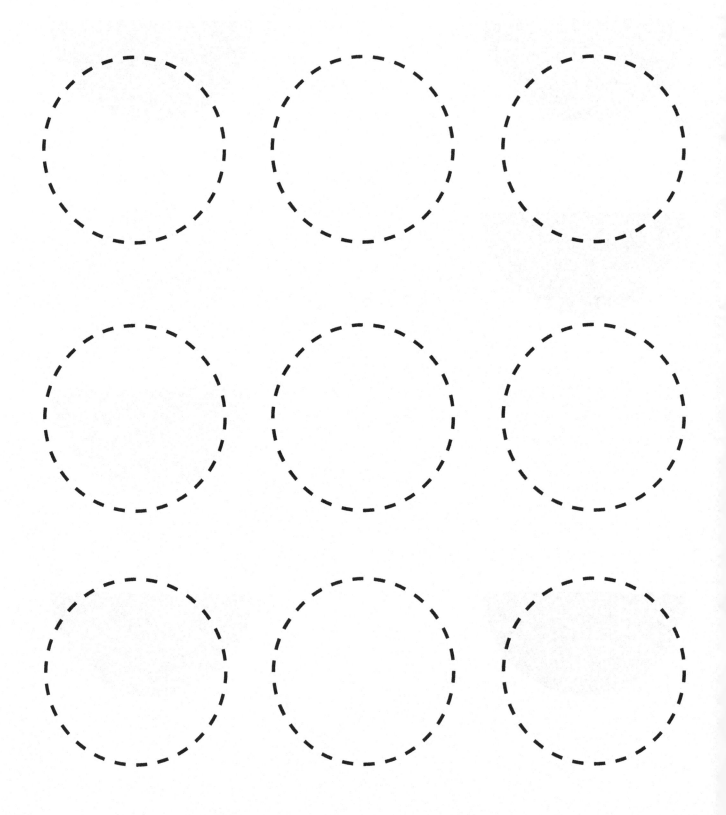

TRACE CIRCLES

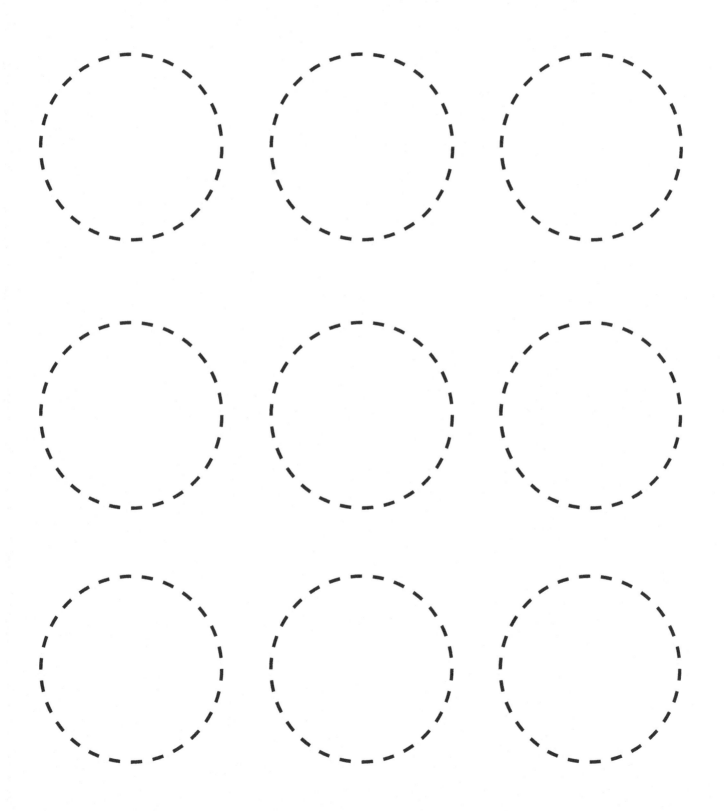

TRACE CIRCLES

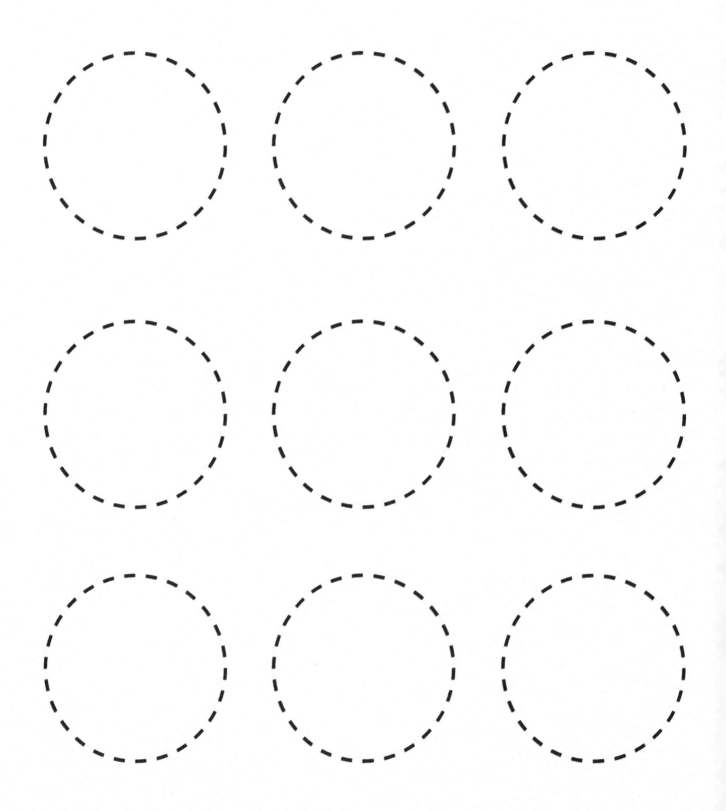

TRACE THE RECTANGLE

TRACE THE RECTANGLE

TRACE THE RECTANGLE

TRACE THE TRIANGLE

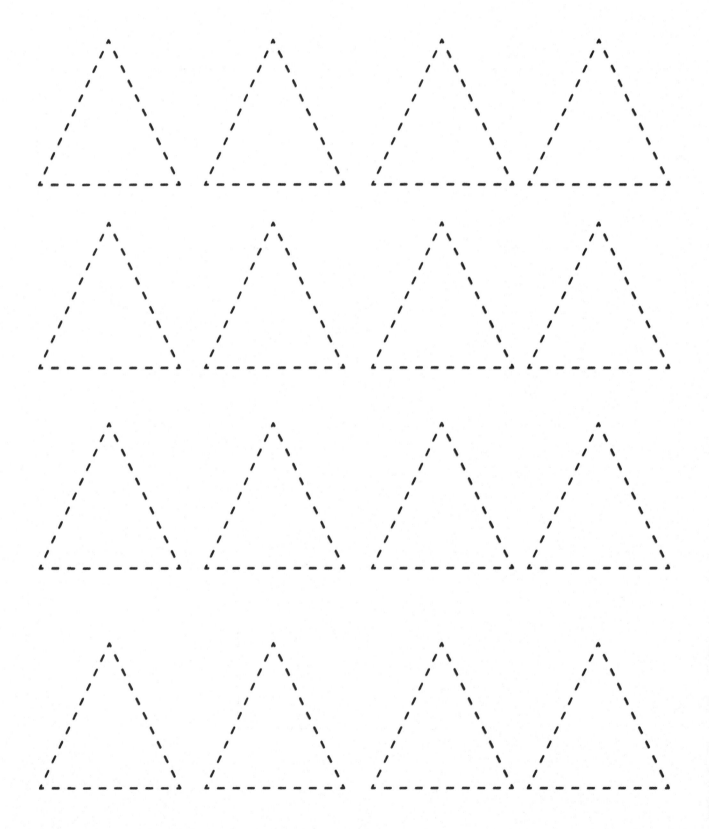

TRACE THE TRIANGLE

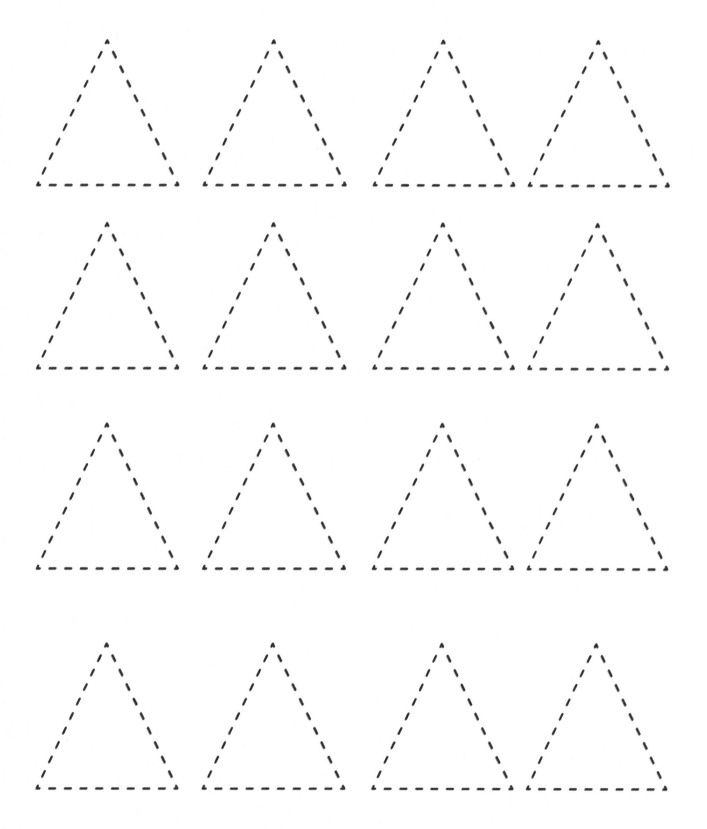

TRACE THE TRIANGLE

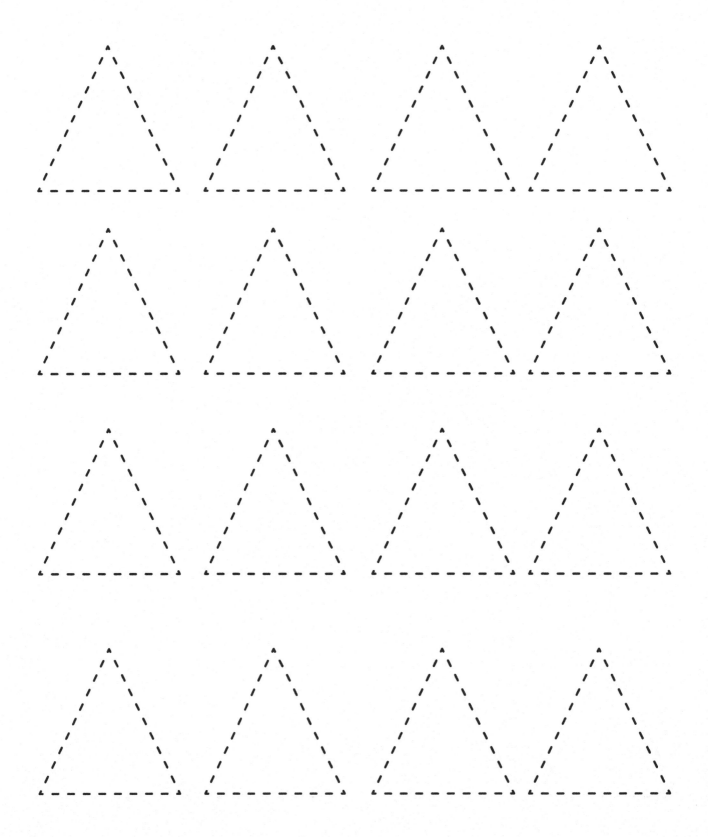

Find And Trace The Shapes

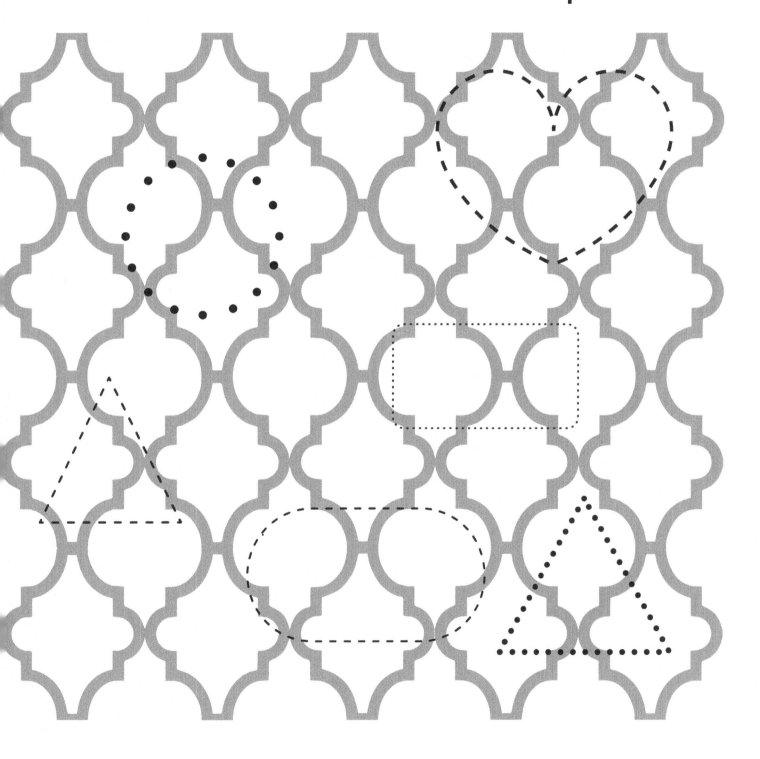

Find And Trace The Shapes

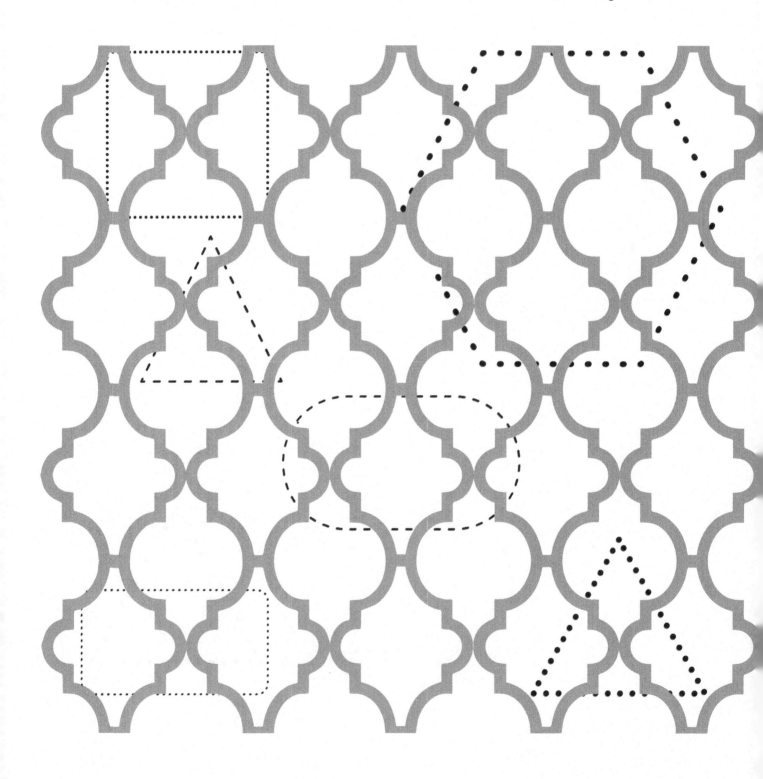

Find And Trace The Shapes

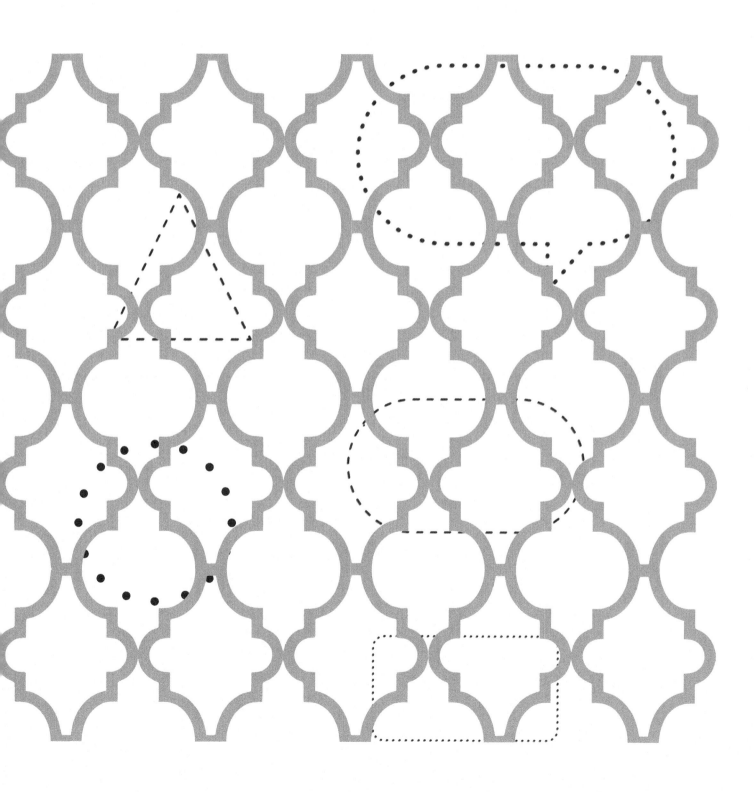

Find And Trace The Shapes

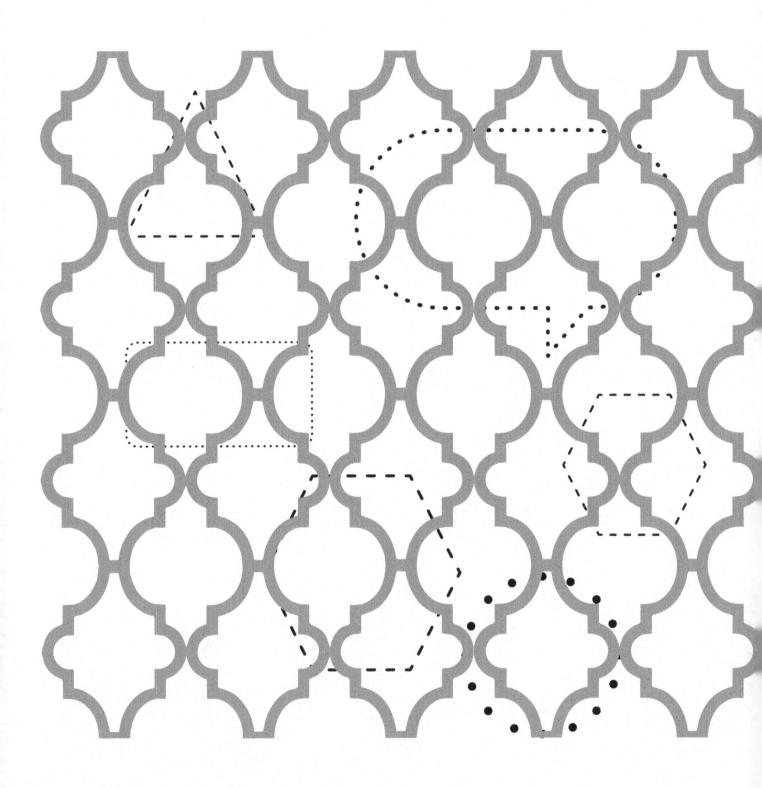

Find And Trace The Shapes

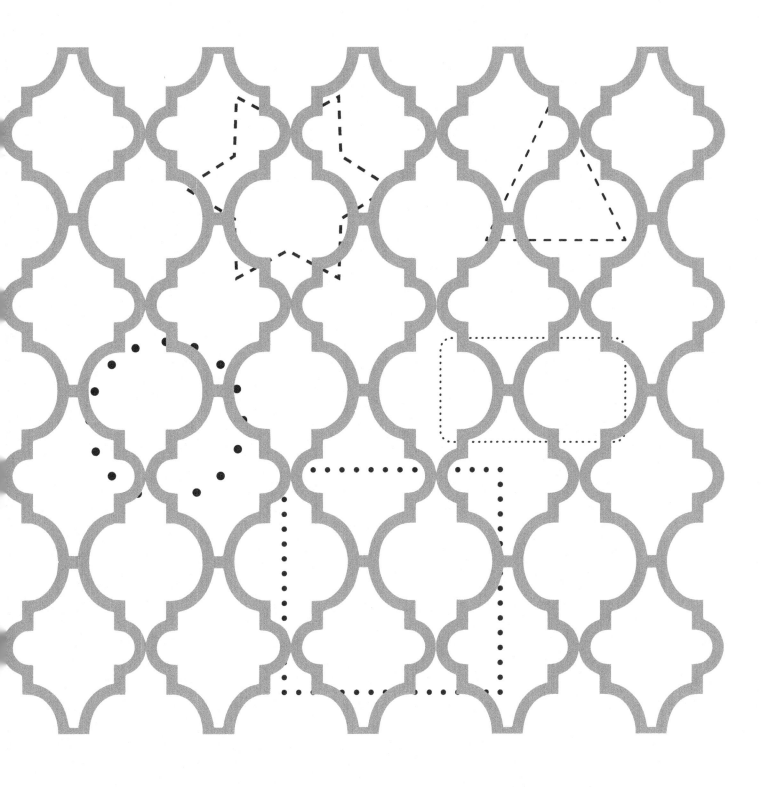

Find And Trace The Shapes

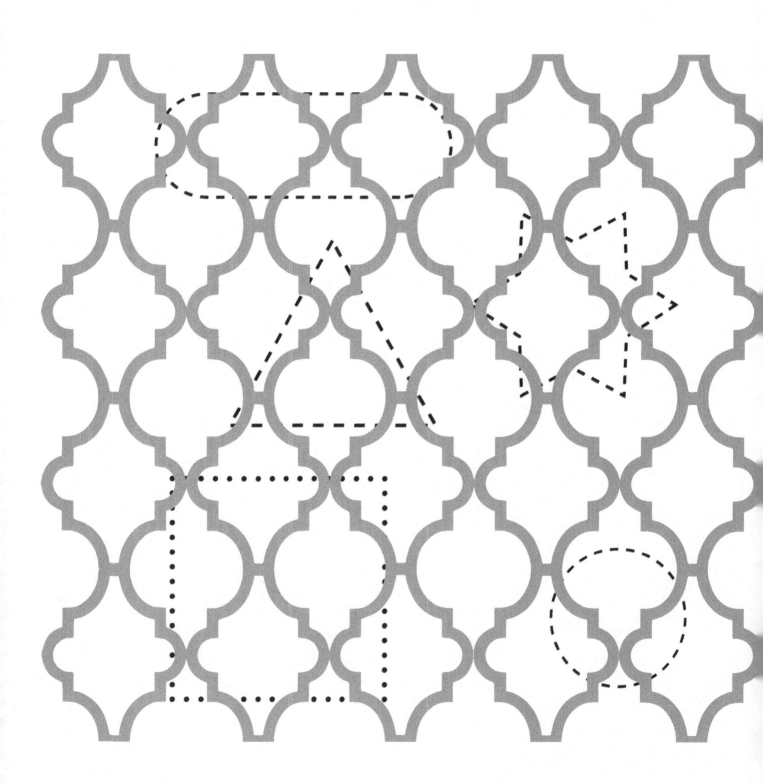

LET'S PLAY SUDOKU

1

			7	8				1
		1	4					2
		7						
2	5						4	8
6					5			
		4	9					
7			1	2	9	8		
				3		7	5	
	8							3

LET'S PLAY SUDOKU
2

4		6	8				9	
		8	6	2			5	4
				1	4			
5							4	8
8		7		3	5			
	9			6		2		3
1							8	
								6

LET'S PLAY SUDOKU
3

					9			3
				4				
6		9	7			4		5
		7					8	
5		4					1	
					6	3	5	
								8
		1	6	9				
4	8		2			1		

LET'S PLAY SUDOKU
4

				5		2	7	1
		8			4			
				2		6	4	
5	3	2			6			
		7	4					9
	5						6	
			7				5	
4	6		2			9	1	

LET'S PLAY SUDOKU
5

		1		9		2		
			6			7	9	
						5		8
				3			7	
		8	4	1				3
	9	3						
	2							
7		5			3		8	
	8	4	5		6			

LET'S PLAY SUDOKU
6

5						1		4
	8	9							
		2		9				3
			8	2				1
						7	4	
					4	3		
6					5		3	
		4	7	8				
	8			4		6	7	

LET'S PLAY SUDOKU

7

4		9						1
	6	2					9	
5			6			3		
							1	
				4				
1			3	2		8		
		5			2	9	7	
6	2						3	
			8		7		5	6

LET'S PLAY SUDOKU
8

			6	8				
	8	3			9		6	
	7					4		1
	3				7			
								4
		9		4		7	2	8
	5	7	1		3			
		8		6	4		7	

Solution 1

5	6	3	7	8	2	4	9	1
8	9	1	4	5	3	6	7	2
4	2	7	6	9	1	3	8	5
2	5	9	3	6	7	1	4	8
6	1	8	2	4	5	9	3	7
3	7	4	9	1	8	5	2	6
7	3	5	1	2	9	8	6	4
1	4	2	8	3	6	7	5	9
9	8	6	5	7	4	2	1	3

Solution 2

4	1	6	8	5	7	3	9	2
3	7	8	6	2	9	1	5	4
9	5	2	3	1	4	8	6	7
5	3	1	2	7	6	9	4	8
6	2	9	4	8	1	7	3	5
8	4	7	9	3	5	6	2	1
7	9	4	5	6	8	2	1	3
1	6	3	7	4	2	5	8	9
2	8	5	1	9	3	4	7	6

SOLUTION 3

2	4	5	1	6	9	8	7	3
8	7	3	5	4	2	6	9	1
6	1	9	7	8	3	4	2	5
3	6	7	9	5	1	2	8	4
5	2	4	8	3	7	9	1	6
1	9	8	4	2	6	3	5	7
9	5	2	3	1	4	7	6	8
7	3	1	6	9	8	5	4	2
4	8	6	2	7	5	1	3	9

SOLUTION 4

3	4	6	8	5	9	2	7	1
2	7	8	6	1	4	3	9	5
1	9	5	3	2	7	6	4	8
5	3	2	1	9	6	7	8	4
6	1	7	4	3	8	5	2	9
9	8	4	5	7	2	1	3	6
7	5	1	9	4	3	8	6	2
8	2	9	7	6	1	4	5	3
4	6	3	2	8	5	9	1	7

SOLUTION 5

8	5	1	3	9	7	2	6	4
4	3	2	6	5	8	7	9	1
9	6	7	2	4	1	5	3	8
2	4	6	8	3	5	1	7	9
5	7	8	4	1	9	6	2	3
1	9	3	7	6	2	8	4	5
6	2	9	1	8	4	3	5	7
7	1	5	9	2	3	4	8	6
3	8	4	5	7	6	9	1	2

SOLUTION 6

5	6	3	2	7	8	1	9	4
8	9	1	4	6	3	5	2	7
4	7	2	5	9	1	8	6	3
3	4	6	8	2	7	9	5	1
2	5	8	1	3	9	7	4	6
7	1	9	6	5	4	3	8	2
6	2	7	9	1	5	4	3	8
9	3	4	7	8	6	2	1	5
1	8	5	3	4	2	6	7	9

SOLUTION 7

4	7	9	2	5	3	6	8	1
3	6	2	4	1	8	7	9	5
5	1	8	6	7	9	3	4	2
2	5	3	7	8	6	4	1	9
7	8	6	9	4	1	5	2	3
1	9	4	3	2	5	8	6	7
8	3	5	1	6	2	9	7	4
6	2	7	5	9	4	1	3	8
9	4	1	8	3	7	2	5	6

SOLUTION 8

2	4	5	6	8	1	9	3	7
1	8	3	4	7	9	5	6	2
9	7	6	5	3	2	4	8	1
8	3	4	2	1	7	6	5	9
7	6	2	8	9	5	3	1	4
5	1	9	3	4	6	7	2	8
4	5	7	1	2	3	8	9	6
3	2	8	9	6	4	1	7	5
6	9	1	7	5	8	2	4	3

You are loved and we appreciate you, and your fight.

TO ALL STROKE SURVIVORS.

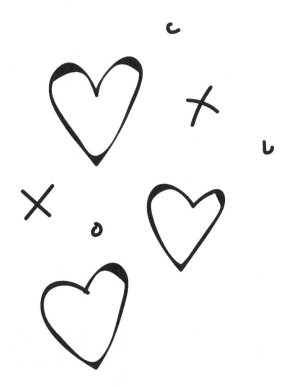

Made in the USA
Las Vegas, NV
28 July 2022

52327375R00057